clean mind,
clean body

DEY ST.
An Imprint of WILLIAM MORROW

clean mind, clean body

A 28-DAY PLAN FOR PHYSICAL, MENTAL, AND SPIRITUAL SELF-CARE

Tara Stiles

This book contains advice and information relating to health care. It should be used to supplement rather than replace the advice of your doctor or another trained health professional. If you know or suspect you have a health problem, it is recommended that you seek your physician's advice before embarking on any medical program or treatment. All efforts have been made to assure the accuracy of the information contained in this book as of the date of publication. This publisher and the author disclaim liability for any medical outcomes that may occur as a result of applying the methods suggested in this book.

FIRST EDITION

Designed by Michelle Crowe
All photos courtesy of the author

Library of Congress Cataloging-in-Publication Data has been applied for.

ISBN 978-0-06-294731-4

20 21 22 23 24   LSC   10 9 8 7 6 5 4 3 2 1

For all the busy people looking for a better way to get it all done and feel better in the process.

I hope this helps.

contents

CLEAN BODY

CLEAN LIVING FOR LIFE

introduction:

ancient wisdom
made new

A healthy mind is the key factor for a healthy body . . .
wellness must include a happy mind.
—His Holiness the 14th Dalai Lama

n many ways, you could say that we are living in the golden age
of wellness. Back when I was growing up in the 1980s and '90s,
you would hear a lot of talk about the importance of eating well
and exercising, but there was a big piece of the conversation missing: few people were talking about mental well-being and the mind-
body connection. That part of the wellness equation was mostly left
out, and mental health just didn't get much attention unless there
was a really serious issue.

Today all that has changed. It is now widely acknowledged in
our culture that the mind and body are interconnected. We openly
discuss our mental health, and many of us maintain practices like
meditation and yoga that draw on ancient wisdom to promote the
mind-body connection. We are living in a time of incredible awareness and opportunity when it comes to wellness. And yet, ironically,

while we understand the mind-body connection intellectually, we are completely out of touch with its application, how to live in a way that facilitates mental and physical balance. We feel burdened by the pressure to appear "well" to the world, documenting our lives on social media, sharing an airbrushed version of reality with the world for validation. We subscribe to the cult of "crazy busy," bragging about our stress and wearing our sleep deprivation as a badge of honor. We throw around buzzwords like "self-care," but we don't understand the true meaning of wellness. Most of us only get serious about tending to our minds and our bodies when we are in crisis—when we feel sick or sluggish, when we are stressed out beyond belief, when we are consumed by anxiety, depression, or mental fog. In search of relief, we commit to the next fad diet, try a new workout, or book a few sessions with a trainer, hoping it will make us feel better. And maybe we do feel better for a while, but it doesn't last.

AS I MAKE THE FINAL EDITS on this book, we find ourselves in the midst of the coronavirus pandemic, and many of us around the world are in lockdown, ordered to stay at home and practice social distancing and not partake in group activities, such as communal meals with friends and in-person exercise classes, to prevent the virus from spreading. During this time, I have been reflecting on how fortunate I am to have the privilege of staying home, feeling grateful that my friends and family are safe, and checking in with them regularly over the phone. Those of us staying at home have the easy job, while medical professionals and other essential workers are out there putting themselves at risk in order to keep us safe. We must recognize that we are being given a once-in-a-lifetime opportunity to take the cue to slow down seriously. If we let this time pass without heeding this call, we will have missed a massive moment for lasting transformation.

It's a good time to reflect on how you are, what your priorities are, and how you spend your time. It's a good time to reflect on what you would do if you could do anything at all. Now is a time of reinvention if you feel stuck. Now is a time of simplification if you feel too busy. Now is a time of peace if you feel anxious. Now is a time to look inside, realign, and point your energy where you truly want to be.

Deep down, what we really want is to be free from the toxic cycle of stress, anxiety, and insecurity. It's uncomfortable to admit how disconnected we have become from our true selves, from our mental, physical, and spiritual health, and from our relationships with others. We want a better way, but we don't know where to begin. And we are addicted to outsourcing our wellness. Instead of jumping on the bandwagon and trying the next quick fix that promises to help us feel better, we need to take a step back. Pause. And hit the reset button.

The ancient practices that many of us now subscribe to as part of "wellness culture" were able to develop on a much different timeline, back when people weren't trying to squeeze so much into a day. Ayurveda, yoga, meditation, and the healing arts arose out of self-study and trial and error by practitioners who shared a common quest to know themselves and to share their knowledge with their communities. What started to take hold in these ancient societies was practical healthcare, a way of maintaining health and well-being as part of daily life, rather than waiting until we are sick to intervene and address health issues. For example, shiatsu, a form of Japanese bodywork based on concepts in traditional Chinese medicine (TCM), was originally practiced in the home between family members as a normalized practice of caring for each other. Can you imagine families doing this together today?

We need to remind ourselves that the power to heal exists in the actual practices, and that these practices live inside of us. The answers are not external. With yoga, change happens when your body comes into harmony with your mind through movement. With meditation, change happens when you quiet your thoughts and connect with a deeper sense of who you are. With Ayurveda, change happens when you get back in touch with nature and the seasons through the foods you prepare and eat. Sure, we can buy products that remind, aid, and inspire us to make positive changes, but none of these things are necessary. True healing is simple, and it starts within. It begins with a decision and a commitment to change.

It's important to keep in mind that these ancient practices are only valuable to us if we can tailor them to fit in with our modern lives and our needs. The challenge for most of us is going from knowing to doing. It's in deciding to take steps to make change in our lives because we desire to feel better, and it's in making these practices work for us, day in and day out.

That is where this book comes in. *Clean Mind, Clean Body* is a 28-day journey that will show you how to use these ancient practices, and some modern ones, to reestablish the mind-body connection in your own life. It is a detox plan for both your mind and your body, intended to set you on the path to healthier, more sustainable habits for life. I'm going to show you how to integrate well-being into every part of your life, and I'm going to guide you through setting clean living goals that I hope will transform your health and your life.

This 28-day journey is divided into four parts, each a weeklong segment that focuses on a particular area of your life and shows you how to hit the reset button on your habits in that area. Week 1 is your Mental Cleanse, because the mind is where it all begins. During this first week we'll focus on recalibrating your habits for better work-life balance and a more sustainable pace of life, as well as reconnecting with yourself and with others. Week 2 is your Spiritual Detox, where we'll focus on reconnecting with your spiritual side, establishing a daily meditation practice, and living with greater intention. Week 3 is Change the Way You Eat, when we'll get into the kitchen and learn to nourish and love our bodies through the lens of Ayurveda and other tested wisdoms. Week 4 is Change the Way You Move, where we'll redefine exercise and shift the way that you think about and relate to your body. Throughout this journey, I'm going to recommend practices and exercises for you to try, based on what has worked for me and for my students. You will want to be sure to also have a blank journal handy as you read this book, for completing the journaling exercises, and for jotting down any other thoughts or insights that come to you.

Clean Mind, Clean Body is a plan for realigning your habits toward serving you and that sets you on a path toward the life you want and how you want to feel. As you embark on this journey, keep in mind that ancient practices like meditation, Ayurveda, and yoga aren't foreign. They live inside of all of us, waiting to be unlocked. True wellness isn't about buying the right products or equipment or achieving a fixed goal like a number on the scale or a number of workouts per week. It's about getting real, committing to change, and confronting the destructive habits that are holding us back. Only then can we begin to meet ourselves halfway and work toward a life where our minds and our bodies exist in harmony.

When I have a day that is going wacky, I try to squeeze in a second shower—not because my body needs to be cleaned, but because I enjoy the experience as a kind of symbolic reset. It could be the middle of the afternoon, but I'll say to myself, "Let's start this day again." This journey I'm going to lead you on in this book is a whole-self reboot that strips backs the layers to reveal the real you. Imagine stepping off the wellness hamster wheel and finally feeling at peace in your body, while living with a deep knowledge of who you are, what you want, and how you want to serve in this world.

Clean Mind, Clean Body is your personal blueprint for realignment, your second shower. We're going to learn ways to nourish the mind, body, and the spirit. We're also going to explore modern updates to ancient practices that can add amazing value to your life, while working toward shedding the habits that limit your potential. Let this journey be a reminder of the wisdom inside of you that is just waiting to be activated, coupled with a giant permission slip to slow down, get back in touch with your senses, and return to the most essential version of yourself. It's time to live and enjoy your best life.

—Tara Stiles,

APRIL 2020

clean
mind

1

hit the reset:

mental detox

Nature does not hurry, yet everything is accomplished.
—Lao Tzu

I f we want to live in harmony and be the best versions of ourselves that we can be—in our careers, to our families, and with our friends—we need to address the body as a whole. And that begins in our minds. Reconnecting our bodies with our minds starts with something that is already inside us: our breath. We breathe all day long without even thinking about it, but most of us aren't activating the true potential of this inner resource. Our breath lives within us, it moves through us, and it sustains us. It is at the root of who we are, beyond our own expectations or the expectations of others, and it connects us with our true potential.

When we are stressed, our breath is the first thing to be affected. When external tension enters our bodies, our breath becomes short and shallow. We literally hold our breath when we are tense, shocked, or afraid. We have all heard that breathing properly is good for us, but we turn our backs on the power of our breath, instead functioning on autopilot and struggling our way through. Tension has become our habit.

I believe in a better way. This lyric from Ben Harper's song "Better Way" is a mantra of mine, and I use it a lot when I'm practicing or teaching yoga. You can't access the full potential of your breath if you are tense and rigid. But it is possible to train yourself to be relaxed and moveable even during times of stress by following the practice outlined on page 11. This exercise will help you focus your attention on your breath, allowing it to flow freely through your lungs and throughout your entire body.

This practice should become part of your routine. Try it first thing in the morning, while you are still in bed and before you do anything else. Try it throughout your day as well, while doing simple tasks like taking a shower, loading the dishwasher, or commuting (unless you are the driver!). The idea is to integrate this technique into your routine during moments of calm, so that it becomes second nature. Then, at tense moments, when you feel stress creeping in, you can also access the technique and use it to keep your breath flowing freely, which will help you to deal with the difficult situation. The goal is to train yourself to be moveable—and to *breathe*—in all situations, to bridge the gap between moments when you feel relaxed and moments when you feel stressed. The stress will not disappear, but by accessing your breath, you can train yourself to react to it more mindfully.

clean mind practice:
Connecting with Your Breath

Tai chi is a type of low-impact, slow-motion exercise based on Chinese martial arts and often described as "meditation in motion." It's a practice that involves a series of graceful movements performed in a slow, focused manner and accompanied by deep breathing. This way of moving focuses on the mind-body connection, and it's beneficial for reducing stress and anxiety, promoting flexibility, and even diving into your creativity.

Practice this simple tai chi exercise to tap into the power of your breath and reduce tension in your body and mind. Once you've mastered this simple practice, you'll be able to do it anytime, anywhere, whenever you feel yourself starting to get anxious or stressed.

1. Sit or stand comfortably. It is important to be comfortable for this exercise, otherwise tension creeps in so easily. Adjust yourself in any way you need to in order to be comfortable. Close your eyes.

2. Soften your body a bit. Relax your knees, your elbows, and your shoulders. Imagine that you are allowing your body to be moved, so that if someone nudged you gently, you would sway like a tree in the wind. Remain soft and moveable. Let yourself exist here, just for a moment.

3. Take a single, deep inhale through your nose. Notice your body lift up and expand in reaction to your inhale. Release a long, easy exhale through your mouth. Notice your body

relaxing downward. Repeat this big inhale and long exhale twice more. Notice your body moving slightly after your breath, following it in response, not at the same time, but being pulled and supported by your breath.

4. Keep your eyes closed. How does your body feel? Softer? Do you feel tension anywhere? Take note. When you are ready, gently open your eyes.

Setting Goals:
How Do You Want to Feel?

Now that you know how to access your breath, let's take stock of where you are right now and where you want to be at the end of your 28-day *Clean Mind, Clean Body* journey. Keep those deep, softening breaths going. No one is judging here. This is simply a structure to set the stage for the new way of living that you are going to try on for size.

Before you start jotting down your goals, remember this, above all else: You are not broken. Say this out loud and write it in your journal in all caps if that helps. You may be here because you have acquired some less-than-ideal habits that have led to some not-so-great results in your life. But guess what? *You* are not your habits. And habits can be changed. Also keep in mind that change is incremental. One small, simple act can have a ripple effect in your day, and in your life, leading to many other good decisions and new habits.

A recent interaction with one of my yoga students illustrates this ripple effect. This student had been in my class every day for a week, and she approached me one day to say that she had something to share. She explained that while there was nothing really "wrong" with her life, she had been feeling disengaged, like she was sort of just going through the motions. But she was excited to tell me that simply by showing up to practice yoga with us every day that week, she was feeling more energy and enthusiasm for other parts of her life, and that her interactions at work, and with her family and friends, were suddenly brighter and more meaningful. The only change she had made was practicing yoga with us every day. She was showing up and taking care of herself.

journal it out:
feel-good goals

Okay, now it's your turn. Grab your journal and a pencil or pen. Ask yourself, "What are my goals for this 28-day journey, rooted in the way that I want to feel during this time?" Keep it simple—eight to ten goals are enough. Remember, these goals should not be about a fixed endpoint that you want to achieve. This is about how you want to feel.

As an example, here are the goals I've set for myself:

I want to have energy when I wake up and feel great during the day.

I want to get sick less often and recover more quickly when I do.

I want to feel more confident.

I want to experience joy more often.

I want to feel connected to my family and friends.

I want to feel at peace and enjoy calm when I am at home.

I want to feel a sense of purpose on a daily basis.

I want to feel like I am continuing to grow and improve in all I do.

The great thing about feeling-based goals is that once you begin to shift your habits and behaviors, you will begin to experience the rewards of your efforts right away!

My decision to become a yoga teacher, a profession that gives me immense joy and that allows me to experience all the feel-good benefits described on page 14 on a daily basis, was not the result of a fixed-endpoint goal that I set for myself. At age twenty-one, after moving to New York City fresh out of a contemporary dance conservatory, where I was introduced to yoga and fell in love with the practice, I thought I was going make my way as a dancer and choreographer. Yoga was a passion of mine, but it was something that I viewed as a personal tool. I didn't imagine spending my life sharing yoga with others.

I was cobbling together an income with dance and choreography gigs, appearances in TV commercials, and modeling jobs, and I was generally happy and having fun, but I also felt a larger sense of disconnection from what I was doing. My schedule was packed, but every job I landed was for the purpose of getting to the next thing. I looked for meaning in each gig and I wasn't finding it, only a race to the next opportunity. At times, the hustle was energizing, and I was grateful to have steady work. But at the same time, I was really running myself ragged and not feeling even close to fully myself. I was always trying to show a side of me that I thought would get the gig without figuring out who I really was or what I really wanted. Occasionally, on one of these gigs, I would mention my passion for yoga to a production assistant, a camera operator, or a makeup artist, and I'd find that I couldn't stop talking excitedly about it.

Eventually, out of all this talk, someone asked me to teach them yoga one-on-one. I agreed, and from that first class I taught, I felt fully myself, and fully alive, in a way I never had before. It wasn't like the other work I was doing, where I had to put on an act, or appear a certain way. I was fully sharing what I was passionate about with another person, and I loved it. My first yoga session led to referrals, and before I knew it, I had a number of private clients.

Occasionally, when someone would ask me what I was doing and I would answer that I was teaching private yoga sessions to people in their homes, I would get a funny look—like things must not be going so well for me. In the circles of dance and people going on auditions in NYC, doing anything else with your time was sort of looked down upon. There was this pressure to constantly be busy with gigs, and if you had free time and let that time slip into other areas of interest, you were on your way out. I hadn't been looking for a way out, but I found myself so happy teaching yoga, and I followed that feeling.

Before discovering my passion for yoga, most of my goals were endpoint based. They were about the destination, rather than the journey. I knew that I needed to earn a certain amount each month to pay my rent and my bills, and I set my goals based on what I needed to earn to pay those bills, with a bit left over for savings. Of course, we all have bills to pay and I'm not suggesting that you should ignore your bills. But my goals weren't inspired, and I had blinders on to the greater possibilities in my life. Once I discovered my passion for teaching yoga, the way I set goals for myself completely changed. My actions became rooted in this new kind of goal setting, based on how I wanted to feel rather than what I wanted to achieve. This was a huge, liberating shift for me. My goal became to feel passion and engagement in all that I did in my life. And that is the way I try to live now.

NOW THAT WE UNDERSTAND the kind of goals that we should be setting for this journey, let's dive right into Week 1, our Mental Detox. We begin with a week devoted to calming and quieting the mind, because without a "clean mind" as our solid foundation, anything else we try to build or achieve will lack stability. Looking ahead, when we embark on Week 2, we will continue cultivating and building on our Week 1 practices. Ideally, each week's practices will have become habit by the time we enter the following week. Week 1 will focus on the following elements:

- *Creating Sanctuary:* Set the stage for transformation by decluttering your home and cultivating harmony in your physical space.

- *Work-Life and Tech-Life Balance:* Set boundaries for a healthier relationship with technology and recalibrate your habits for work-life balance and a more sustainable pace of life.

- *Nurturing Relationships:* This week is about reconnecting with yourself and rekindling your relationships with others.

CREATING SANCTUARY

The way that you feel inside, your "internal ecosystem," is largely influenced by your external environment. This is why clearing out and cleaning your home is the first stage of Clean Mind. I'm sure you've noticed that when your kitchen is a mess, you are more likely to reach for junk food than you are to cook something healthy. Or that if there is a giant pile of laundry on the floor of your bedroom, you are less likely to jump out of bed and want to do something productive. Our physical environment affects our mental state.

Cleaning house is about more than checking off the chores and taking out the trash. It's about contemplating how you want to *feel* in your space. Your home serves certain practical functions: it is a place to stay safe and warm and protected from the elements; it is a place where you relax, sleep, and cook and eat your meals. But the quality of these actions—resting, sleeping, eating, etc.—is affected by the care and attention you put into your physical space. In order to achieve mental clarity and balance, we often need to shed the unnecessary, extraneous things in our physical lives. By cleaning, we also cultivate gratitude for the way that our homes and the objects in them serve us and bring us comfort. In yoga, we often talk about meditation as "peeling the onion of the self." I like to think of cleaning house as peeling the onion of our physical environment.

We're at a cultural tipping point with all the excess stuff in our homes. We ended up here with mostly good intentions, maybe buying things we didn't really need because they were on sale, or hanging on to items because of their sentimental value. But clutter in our homes has the effect of making us feel overwhelmed, disconnected from nature and our environment, and spiritually exhausted. Practices like minimalism, tidying, donating, recycling, and upcycling have suddenly become cool because we're realizing that another pair of jeans isn't going to make us happy, but crafting a pair of old jeans into a rug or donating them gives us a more enriching feeling.

"Decluttering" may be a trend, but the practice itself is nothing new. It is the resurgence of ancient wisdom. Feng shui is the ancient Chinese art of placement designed to create harmony and balance between our surrounding environments (our homes) and the elements of nature. Feng shui is based on the idea that chi (energy or life force) flows through all things, and that there is always a shifting balance between the Taoist principles of yin (feminine energy) and yang (masculine energy) in our environments, as well as the five elements—wood, fire, earth, metal, and water. Feng shui involves organizing and placing certain objects in positions in your home to encourage the flow of energy from one room to the next, and to promote well-being, prosperity, and beauty in the home.

The practice of feng shui can be quite complex, and I'm not going to get into all the details here. But I am going to recommend a very simple practice based on feng shui that promotes harmony and energy flow in your home. According to feng shui, the simple practice of sweeping and clearing your front entryway creates positive flow and promotes well-being. Your front door is very important in feng shui, as it is where anyone enters your home. Instead of having the energy to race up a flight of stairs, or straight to your kitchen, or to whatever room is next to your front door when you come in, you can slow down the energy by adding a mirror, a rug, or a piece of art in your entryway. These mindful and beautiful additions give you and your guests a reason to pause and reflect when entering.

Making Space for How You Want to Feel

When I bring people together for a yoga experience, it is incredibly important that the space we are working in is clean and harmonious. When I'm leading an event in a new space, I always show up early, before any of my students arrive, so I have time to get to know the space, clean up, and organize. I don't leave this to the cleaning crew, and if there are cleaning people on staff, I take pleasure in helping them. For me, picking up trash and sweeping the floor isn't someone else's job if I want to fill that room with the best possible energy. Neither is leaving the room better than I found it when the class is finished. From a practical standpoint, cleaning the space also helps me get to know the environment I'm in. I learn all kinds of useful things while cleaning a yoga studio—like where the light is coming from, where the exits and the bathrooms are, and where possible distractions might be coming in from outside the room—so that I can be fully present when I am teaching. This cleaning ritual began in my professional life, and it has extended into my personal life.

I am not naturally an organized person. I will confess that it usually feels like a heroic effort to make my bed in the morning. If I'm not careful, I will end up with piles of clothes on the bathroom floor, and when guests are coming over, I stuff everything I don't want them to see into various closets. These are my tendencies and habits, but I don't beat myself up for them. I know that they are changeable, and that I'm not stuck with them. I do my best to notice when I'm making a mess and, more important, why I'm making the mess. Usually it's because I'm in a rush and feeling distracted. Noticing that I'm feeling off is inspiration for me to make time to organize. For me, it's not about keeping a pristine home and trying to be perfect. It's about staying in the process and always being interested in and working toward improvement. I used to believe that cleaning and organizing was for people who had loads of free time, and was unattainable for busy people. A mess was something to deal with or outsource. But the more I dove into the process of organizing, the more I realized the process is essential to my well-being. When my home is organized, I feel like I have more time in the day. The same applies for the spaces we spend time in outside the home. Whether we're at work, at school, or in the car, maintaining an organized space creates harmony and fosters creativity and progress.

During meditation, when you notice that your mind is wandering, and that you are moving away from focusing on your breath, you have a clear choice: you can keep letting your thoughts wander, or you can guide yourself back to your breath. The same goes for your physical space. When you notice that pile of dirty laundry on the floor of your room, you have a choice: you can close the bedroom door and pretend that everything's fine, or you can grab that laundry and throw it in your washing machine or hamper! I focus on how I want to feel and how good it feels in the rest of my life to have an organized closet. It sounds a bit silly that picking up a pile of clothes from the floor can give you better head-space for creativity, but there really is a strong connection. Because I love my work so much, I see that pile and remind myself that I will have access to my creativity if I pick it up. When you focus on how you want to feel, it's easy to organize with joy instead of dread.

Our habits are connected to the way we feel inside, our internal ecosystem. If my closet is messy, I know that I will feel mentally un-settled. But if I am aware of my tendency to let my closet get messy, and the mental effects of that mess, I can empower myself instead of beating myself up for being a "messy closet person." I know this habit is not serving me, and I can make a change. Yoga and medita-tion have taught me that I can shift my habits through consistent practice. When I walk into a yoga studio and tidy before teaching a class, I feel harmony and balance that comes as a result, and that will set the tone for the class. Cleaning house follows the same prin-ciples. Cleaning my closet may not be what I naturally prioritize, but I make it a practice because I knew that it promotes balance and harmony in my home and in my mind. I also notice that when I be-gin my day by getting up early, meditating, and sipping warm water with lemon, making my bed and tidying my closet feels easier. One good habit leads to another!

Cleaning with Kids: How to Bring in Play

Cleaning my closet may not ever "spark joy," to quote Marie Kondo. But when it comes to cleaning with my three-year-old daughter, Daisy, it's quite the opposite. When Daisy is finished playing with her toys, we make tidying a game. It turns out that toddlers as young as one or two love to help clean up! Their actual cleaning skills may not be great at first, but that is beside the point. The idea is to get them involved from a young age in order to build good habits as they get older. While we tidy, Daisy and I sing the popular children's song "Cleanup Song," which we learned from *Dora the Explorer*, and sometimes she even starts the song herself. This practice makes cleaning up part of play, and Daisy takes pride in having her things clean and organized. I've even noticed that when we are at the park, she will pick up trash and look for the nearest garbage can, all on her own. I could have never predicted that this would be the result of our cleanup time together. Watching Daisy has taught me that cleaning shouldn't be an act that we compartmentalize as "not fun!" This is something that all of us, kids and adults, can and should embrace.

Make tidying a sacred, daily ritual in your home, and you may actually find yourself looking forward to it! I personally love researching places close to me that accept donations of gently used clothing and furniture. For me, the dread of cleaning and organizing disappears when I think about how things we've outgrown are being used and loved by someone else.

OKAY, IT'S TIME TO GET TO IT! The following are a series of practices for cleaning your space. This is about physically cleaning your space, but the reward is about so much more than a dust-free floor.

House Cleanse

You should make it a habit to do a deep clean of your entire home once a season. It is an incredibly freeing and cathartic experience. And you don't have to feel like Cinderella toiling away—engage the other members of your household to share the work. Designate a day when everyone is available to clean together, as this will lighten the load and allow you to gain a shared appreciation for your space. As mentioned, little ones love to clean! Don't bother with toy brooms and cleaning tools for your kids—let them use the real thing. It's fun to see how much pride Daisy takes in sweeping up piles and gathering dust bunnies from hard-to-reach places like under the bed and couch!

A sustainable, environmentally friendly way to clean is to cut up old T-shirts and towels to make rags, rather than using and throwing away tons of paper towels. It's easy to wash and reuse your homemade rags, and they generally hold up better and clean surfaces more effectively than paper towels do.

You can also make your own nontoxic cleaning products at home. This is cheaper than using store-bought products, better for the environment, and better for you and your family. Here are some simple recipes for nontoxic cleaning products:

All-Purpose Cleaner

1 cup water
1 cup distilled white vinegar
1 or 2 drops essential oil of your choice (optional; I like
    to use peppermint- or lavender-scented oils)
Lemon or orange rind (optional)

Combine all the ingredients in a reusable glass spray bottle. Shake and use as needed.

Stovetop and Refrigerator Cleaner

¼ cup baking soda
1 quart warm water

Combine the baking soda and warm water in a glass jar. Screw the lid on tightly, shake, and use as needed.

Glass Cleaner

2 cups water
½ cup distilled white vinegar
¼ cup rubbing alcohol
1 or 2 drops essential oil of your choice (optional)

Combine all the ingredients in a reusable glass spray bottle. Shake and use as needed.

clean mind practice:
Meditation for a Healing Space

Before you begin cleaning—particularly if tidying up is a challenge for you and you don't consider yourself naturally neat and organized—try this simple meditation. It will help you clear your mind and honor the space you will be cleaning.

1. Sit comfortably. Close your eyes and pay attention to your breath. Enjoy your body lifting in response to your inhale. Notice your body relaxing as you exhale. Stay with this feeling for a moment.

2. Now imagine how you want your space to feel: peaceful, calm, inspiring, creative, or whatever adjective comes to mind. When a word enters your mind, let it stay there for a moment. You can repeat the word in your mind or simply stay with the feeling that it brings you.

3. Continue to breathe deeply for a few more moments, and when you're ready, open your eyes.

Closet Cleanse

I recommend doing a good closet cleanse once a season, whenever you are preparing to shift your wardrobe from winter to spring, from spring to summer, from summer to fall, etc. The idea is to clear out all the stuff in your closet that is taking up space and no longer serving you, like that fifteen-year-old sweater that you never wear, those dresses that you don't love anymore, or that pair of jeans that holds some sort of unhealthy diet motivation over you. Your closet cleanse could take a couple of hours or a couple of days, depending on how deeply your drawers are stuffed. Once you get through your first epic cleanse, doing this once a season gets easier and easier.

When I first got into this habit, I was surprised by how much easier it became to get dressed on a daily basis, to make use of the pieces in my closet, and to pack for trips. Knowing what you have, and only having items in your closets that you actually wear and love, makes a huge difference.

Tidying guru Marie Kondo recommends taking everything out of your drawers and closet and putting it all in a big pile on the floor or on your bed. I've tried this, and while I appreciate the value of a kick-start, this practice is a bit too extreme and overwhelming for me. Instead, I like to go through one drawer or one part of my closet at a time and put whatever items I don't use from just that drawer or part of my closet in a pile on the floor. My rule is that anything I haven't worn or used in the past year, and that doesn't hold strong sentimental value for me, goes on the floor. This way of gradually decluttering allows me to do things in chunks during the day when I have time. Closet cleaning becomes a part of my daily practice just like meditation and yoga.

Once I have that pile of things that are no longer serving me, I divide it into three categories: "repurpose," "give away," and "thrift." Things like old T-shirts, socks with holes in them, and old scarves go in the "repurpose" pile to be used as rags for cleaning or for arts-and-crafts projects with Daisy. Items that are still in great condition but that I just don't wear anymore go into the "give away" pile, to be given to family members or friends who might be into them or to donate to a local charity. I put particularly expensive or trendy items into the "thrift" pile, to be taken to a local thrift or consignment shop and resold. Familiarize yourself with thrift shops and organizations that accept donations in your neighborhood, and find out what types of items they accept before you go so you don't end up being sent away with your big bag of stuff. There are even retailers now that accept clothing donations for recycling, which I think is incredibly cool!

Make Your Bed

Do this every morning! Making the bed seems like such a small, inconsequential thing. But if you are not in the habit of making your bed, adding this practice to your routine can have surprising effects. I used to skip making the bed in the morning, thinking it was a waste of time—I was just going to mess it all up again that night, right? During this period of my life when I wasn't making the bed, I remember also feeling pretty scattered during the day, never fully completing a task before moving on to the next one. When I started making my bed daily, I found that I gained more focus, clarity, and appreciation for the things I had in my life. Making your bed in the morning sets the tone for your day, as it is part of respecting yourself and showing gratitude for your space. Washing and changing your sheets and pillowcases every two weeks is another good practice. So is switching from heavier bedding in the winter to lighter bedding in the spring as a way to align yourself with the energy of the seasons and improve your overall well-being.

Similar to cleaning out your closet, seeing what you really have in your kitchen pantry can be revealing and a bit scary! Chances are, you have loads of expired items on your shelves, multiples of products you tend to repurchase, and piles of things you will be surprised to find stashed away. When I started getting serious about decluttering my kitchen cabinets, I realized I pick up a jar of peanut butter and a jar of coconut oil on just about every grocery store trip. I had so many that it was shocking! After clearing and organizing, I know what I have, I can see everything more clearly, and I am inspired to cook with fresh ingredients regularly. Now I actually keep my spices all lined up in glass canisters, and when I see them, I get excited to sauté some veggies! So let's roll up our sleeves and take a good, sobering look at what's on our pantry shelves. The benefits of cleaning out your pantry are exponential for your well-being, I promise.

Remove all the items from your pantry and cupboards first, and line everything up on your counter. Weed out expired items and throw them away, remembering to empty and recycle the containers they come in whenever possible. If you have multiples of nonperishable items or items you know you won't use, consider donating them to a local food pantry. Return the things you know you want to keep and those that you use on a regular basis to your pantry and store them grouped by type—pastas and grains go on one shelf, canned goods on another, boxed snacks and crackers on another, etc.

WORK-LIFE AND TECH-LIFE BALANCE

A number of years ago, things really began to pick up for me professionally. Strala Yoga, the studio we started in 2008, was expanding into a global collection of Guides and studios. I was involved in several high-profile partnerships that were broadening my reach. In many ways, this was a good thing. I had established myself as a yoga teacher for many years and momentum was starting to pick up. Magazines and newspapers were covering my work and our community often. I was traveling all over the world to give talks and teach yoga classes. I was wrapped up in the excitement of it all, on a roller coaster of weekly international flights and back-to-back events. This was everything I'd ever wanted, right? Not exactly. It was impossible to be fully present in anything that I did because I was always thinking ahead and trying to plan for the next big project. I felt a constant, barely manageable level of stress. At night I would get into bed, and instead of winding down with a book or an evening meditation (as a yoga teacher should!), I would frantically try to organize my schedule for the next day, and answer emails and texts from everyone in different time zones. Often, if I couldn't sleep, I would get out of bed and hop on a chat with a friend or co-worker in a different time zone to talk about a studio or partnership to occupy my mind instead of calming down.

During this period, I felt like my body was wired, literally buzzing and unable to switch off. My shoulders were full of knots and I was physically on edge and jumpy. Ironically, I was contractually obligated by a number of the companies I was working with to post on Instagram about my supposedly fabulous, healthy lifestyle and tag their brands in my posts. I was barely holding it together, but at the same time I worried about having enough cool content to post on social media each day.

Additionally, despite feeling that my real life wasn't nearly as glamorous as the version I posted on Instagram, I found myself addicted to the cycle of validation that comes with sharing your life on social media. I needed that dopamine hit from the likes and comments that would flood in after I posted something. Without that rush, I often found myself alone in a hotel room on a business trip, feeling empty and depressed. There is considerable scientific research now emerging to explain the depleting effects of social media—effects that I was experiencing directly—and researchers are finding that there is a direct correlation between depression and increased social media use, particularly for those who are predisposed to depression. But this part of my life took place before a lot of this research had come out, and I felt pretty alone in my struggle.

I had separated from my husband, Mike, thinking that everything would somehow be fine if I was on my own and free to move at an even faster pace. During the stress of our separation, I ran myself even more ragged, all the while telling myself I was doing better than ever. This way of living was not sustainable for me, and I inevitably hit a breaking point. I remember the moment distinctly: I was on a plane that had just landed and the flight attendant was shaking my shoulders to wake me up and asking me if I was okay. I was completely disoriented, confused as to where I was and why I was there. I eventually realized that I had just flown from Tokyo to LA and had slept the entire flight. I'd thought I was supposed to be in San Francisco the next day for an event, and I was about to run to catch my connecting flight when I realized I had gotten the date wrong and had a day to spare. With nowhere to go, I checked myself into a hotel in LA and slept more. No one knew where I was, and I took the time to hide out. I realized I needed to slow down. There had been several other moments like this one, but I'd ignored them. Change was necessary, but instead I had powered on. But this time, I knew that I needed to listen to what my body, my mind, and the universe were telling me.

Toward the beginning of my mile-a-minute, keep-as-busy-as-possible, hide-behind-your-work period, I had experienced a trauma that I'd pushed under the rug, big-time: I had a miscarriage. It all began when I was in Moscow for an event and told Mike to meet me in Paris afterward for a couple of days. I told him that we'd get pregnant, and then head back to NYC. We stayed at a romantic hotel with great food and had a nice time walking around the city. I knew with all of myself that I would get pregnant at this time, and I did. A few weeks later I took a pregnancy test to confirm what I already knew. We decided to keep it a secret at first, as I had several friends who were having a hard time getting pregnant at the time. At about eight weeks along, Mike and I were shooting a project together, a yoga class that I was leading with three of my friends in the class. I led them to roll up from relaxation and sit comfortably. That was the moment I started bleeding. I finished the shot and headed off to the bathroom, trying not to show my concern to anyone. There was a lot of blood. Worried that stopping short that day would cost the production a lot of money, I continued with the shoot. I kept my secret to myself and didn't even tell Mike until the end of the shoot day. We headed home and started rationalizing that it wasn't a problem, that it could just be spotting, but we both knew better. I saw my doctor the next day and she confirmed that I'd miscarried. And I didn't tell anyone.

Miscarriage is incredibly common, but it's not talked about much. There is unwarranted shame around it. What if it had been my fault? Had I been too active? Had I done something wrong? The stress swirled. I kept going. I taught my classes as if nothing was wrong. A friend brought her new baby into the studio to meet us on the day I was experiencing the most physical pain and bleeding from the miscarriage; I held the baby. On another day, I got a massive migraine, a side effect of miscarriage, but still powered through the day, barely able to see straight. The physical symptoms were rough, but brief. The emotional turmoil lasted years before it turned into a breakdown. Mike and I never really talked through what had happened. He let me stay busy, and I didn't bring it up. We watched several of our friends get pregnant and didn't discuss how that affected us. I threw myself deep into my work and farther away from everything else until I convinced myself my marriage was the problem.

I hesitated to share my experience, feeling guilty because many women have stress and are dealing with difficult situations. Who was I to complain? On the outside, everything in my life looked great. On the inside, it was dark and lonely. After many months of avoiding the pain and the loss, followed by years of personal work reprioritizing what is important to me, I was finally able to heal. My process included lots of quality time and deep conversations with Mike, and unapologetic self-care. Now that I am on the other side of this storm, with a healthy daughter whom I adore, a mended marriage and better communication with Mike, and a career I am satisfied with, I finally feel comfortable sharing this story. Not because I believe the details of my life are particularly interesting or unique, but because the lessons I've learned may be useful to someone else going through a stressful time.

Mike and I got back together shortly after my LA wake-up call and decided to support each other more, particularly when it came to talking about how we feel, how we want to spend our time, and how we want to live. We finally talked about the pain of the miscarriage that we experienced individually. After we were back on more solid ground in our relationship, we decided that we were ready to try for a baby again. I knew that I really had to get serious about slowing down and taking care of myself. I'll admit that my habit of moving too fast and doing too much was still there, although not as persistent. This was going to take work.

As a way to manage my stress and boost my fertility, I continued regular shiatsu sessions with my friend Sam Berlind. Shiatsu is an ancient Japanese healing practice that uses acupressure to correct energy imbalances in the body. A shiatsu practitioner uses their hands to lean into the energy pathways, known as meridians, in the recipient's body, in order to trigger a response that restores balance in the body. Shiatsu isn't like massage, where muscles are manipulated according to the receiver's preference or in response to muscle soreness. Shiatsu involves sustained pressure along the body's meridians. Different meridians are targeted for different issues. A shiatsu pressure point that many people know of for relieving seasickness or dizziness is the middle of the inside of the wrists. You may have seen someone on a boat wearing a bracelet that targets this pressure point. The goal of shiatsu is to activate meridians that need attention so the body can react and come into balance. Shiatsu is a great practice for overall well-being and is often used for treatment of a variety of health issues.

Sam began our first session with a simple question: "How are you feeling?" In response, I started to sweat and my heart raced, and I blurted out, "I'm fine, everything is fine!" Sam could see right through me. He had me lie down with a weighted pillow resting on my belly and breathe deeply, an exercise that helps you to focus on your breath, directing it toward the pillow, and then breathe more deeply, with the effect of reducing anxiety. When Sam began acupressure, he focused on points on the insides of my ankles that align with the reproductive system, and the sensation was intense! With shiatsu, when part of you is out of balance, you will feel a strong sensation along the meridian that corresponds to that function. That sensation is your body's cue to come back into balance. Shiatsu is a bit like adjusting your body's circuitry, so that energy can flow more easily through your body and bring you back into balance.

After a few months of working with Sam, I got serious about slowing down—out of respect for myself, my well-being, and my future. After each session with him, I could feel my body telling me that slowing down was the best way forward for me. I realized I had a choice about the way I was living: I could race right back into my day after these sessions, or I could change what wasn't working for me. I started to modify many of my habits, like drinking coffee all day long (which made me anxious!), saying yes to everything, even when I was overextended, and staying up late into the night on my computer worrying about it all. I started taking daily walks to clear my mind, without my phone. I loosened my grip on the addictive feedback loop of social media and instead set rules for a healthier, sustainable relationship with sharing online. I

clean mind practice:
Deep Belly Breathing

Try this simple breathing technique that Sam taught me to help your body and mind slow down.

1. Lie on your back on a soft but firm surface, like a carpet or yoga mat on the floor. Adjust yourself so that you are comfortable here.

2. Place a pillow on your lower belly. Close your eyes and take 10 long, deep breaths, focusing on filling your low belly, rather than your chest or rib cage, with air.

3. Allow yourself to rest here and relax for a few moments. When you're ready, gently remove the pillow and slowly bring yourself up to a seated position. It's just as important to take your time as you come out of this exercise as it is to work on breathing deeply during it. Don't hurry to come out.

got focused about my self-care time and created a daily meditation and yoga routine that I stuck to. I also began taking the time to prepare nourishing meals at home. I reflected honestly on whether my actions and choices were leading me in the direction I wanted to go. As a yoga teacher, I was instructing my students to find ease, softness, and balance in their own lives, but I wasn't living the example of my teachings.

I made simplifying my life a priority. I streamlined my local business from nonstop classes, workshops, and trainings to a refreshing welcome center with pop-up classes and a manageable training schedule. When I traveled for work, I started taking longer trips, building in time to enjoy the people and places I was visiting, rather than squeezing in as many back-to-back events as possible. After about a year of living this way, I found that I was feeling calm, centered, balanced, and expansive. Eventually, I got pregnant with Daisy, and life became about more than just planning for myself.

After having Daisy, I felt a need to slow down even more. It is important for me to spend a significant amount of time with her, so I adjusted my work life accordingly. I'm lucky to have Mike as a partner in parenting as well as in our work, and we have found a parenting balance that works for us. There is very little downtime when you have little ones, and keeping up a self-care routine can be challenging. Certain things are just not realistic when you have kids, like getting great sleep when you have a newborn or spending lots of solo time meditating. But once I had Daisy, I discovered a new balance in which self-care practices I could let fade away for the time being and which ones were nonnegotiable. These days, with a toddler, my nonnegotiables are daily meditation and yoga, even if it's only 10 minutes some days. Preparing nourishing meals and giving myself time to explore my hobbies and interests, usually in the form of reading a book on East Asian arts before bed, are also

enlisting an energy practitioner

If you are considering enlisting the help of a professional energy practitioner in your journey toward balance, like I did when I reached out to Sam Berlind, it's important to find the right fit. Whether you are looking for a shiatsu practitioner, an acupuncturist, or another type of healer, ask friends and other people you know and trust for recommendations. Hearing about a practitioner's capabilities from someone you trust is much better than googling "healers near me."

When you book your first session, think of it as an opportunity to feel out whether you are comfortable working with that particular practitioner. They should take a medical history, ask you about your overall health and well-being, and take the time to listen to your answers and respond thoughtfully. If anything about the person's approach or the treatment itself feels off to you, don't hesitate to speak up, and don't force yourself to go back for another session if you aren't feeling it, and feel empowered to leave the session midway if you're uncomfortable.

Don't add to your stress financially. A good practitioner will rely on repeat clients and referrals and shouldn't ask you to pay something outlandish. If the cost is a concern or stress for you, ask the practitioner what your payment options are, and if they have a sliding scale. Good ones will. You may also find, after doing some research, that your insurance plan or FSA will cover some of the costs of an energy practitioner.

important. It's not dramatic, but it has been useful to realize what I can let go of and what I need to keep in my routine for different phases of life. When it came to work, projects that I wasn't excited about faded out of my life and space opened up for the things I truly cared about.

Slowing down had always been my biggest fear, as if everything would fall apart if I gave up the crazy-busy thing. But it turned out to have the exact opposite effect. As soon as I slowed down and let go of the things that were no longer priorities, my work life and my personal life both became much more stable. This was incredibly surprising to me. What I discovered, and what I hope you will discover, is that slowing down is really a process of getting to know yourself and what your needs are for different phases of life, and being open to change.

This more balanced way of living is not an endpoint for me. Instead, I think of it as a new road that I am walking on. My work is still important, but it has become a journey that complements the rest of my life, rather than taking over my entire life. I set boundaries between my work and the rest of my life, and make time for my passions and for the people who matter to me, and these things fuel who I am professionally and creatively.

Work-Life Balance: Is It Really Possible?

The answer is yes, but you need to set boundaries. Whether you work full-time or part-time, from home or in an office, in a creative profession or in a more buttoned-up corporate environment, you need to draw lines between your work life and the rest of your life. These should be designated blocks of time during your day, and your week, when you are truly off duty. Once you set these boundaries, there will of course be exceptions, times when it's necessary to answer a work email or make a call after your designated work hours. We all know how easy it can be to let the lines between work and life blur, checking and answering emails at all hours of the day, night, and weekend. It takes real awareness and conscious choices to set boundaries for yourself. But establishing healthy boundaries will set you on the path toward achieving your larger goals.

On the following pages are some of my personal practices for establishing healthy work-life boundaries. These are the practices that work for me; you may want to adopt them for yourself, or modify them to fit your needs and your schedule. My main recommendation for implementing these practices is to start small. If you get extreme with it right away, you'll probably end up throwing in the towel and hiding under the covers and scrolling through your phone before you know it. Start with just one change—like no phone or email after a certain time at night—and stick with it, and you will find that it has an amazing ripple effect in your life, sparking other new, healthy habits. Then build on this one change as you go.

Morning Yoga and Meditation

No matter what my day has in store, my morning yoga, followed by meditation, is nonnegotiable. For me, this part of my day is more important than a shower. Sometimes it happens right when I wake up, and sometimes it happens midmorning, after I make breakfast for everyone. I let myself be flexible on exactly when, but it has to happen sometime in the morning before I start my day, and it has to last for at least 10 minutes. I know that I can find at least those 10 minutes, even on the most hectic day. On busy days, I'll set a timer for 10 minutes and let myself move however feels best for me, finishing with a short meditation. On days when I have more time, I don't worry about the timer, and I'll continue for 20 minutes to an hour. I

clean mind practice:
Meditation for Work-Life Harmony

This is a great practice to incorporate during your morning meditation, particularly during periods of professional stress when you need to return to your center and regain balance. Be sure to have a journal or notebook handy for this practice.

1. Sit comfortably. Take a moment to listen to your breath. Take notice of how you feel. Are there particular thoughts and emotions that are coming up for you this morning? Does your mind race immediately toward work tasks, or does that give you a feeling of dread? As you breathe in and out, you are going to set an intention for the kind of balance you want to achieve between your work and the rest of your life. Think back to a time when your career and your personal life were in balance and at peace. Picture what this looked like and remember how it felt. If you haven't yet experienced work-life balance, imagine what this would look and feel like in your life today. Stay with this image.

2. Return to your breath. Take a moment to inhale and exhale deeply. Notice how you feel. Take a moment to sit calmly before you open your eyes.

3. Now pick up your journal and jot down a description of the kind of work-life harmony that you just envisioned. Write down any experiences and feelings that came to mind during the meditation. Think about how this envisioning practice can lead you to make some simple changes in the way you work and live.

recommend doing the Energizing Yoga Flow on page 208, followed by this morning meditation practice, one that I love.

Office Hours

Because I work for myself, and I work from home, from an office, from planes, and from pretty much any other place, I have to create my own boundaries and make my own office hours. It would be easy for me to stay up way too late working and then pick up where I left off first thing in the morning, but knowing myself, I've created a few rules. In the morning I don't check email or do anything work-related until after I've done my 10 minutes of yoga and meditation. If something is truly urgent, I'll make an exception, but I generally keep this boundary. Same goes for the evenings. I'll often work a bit after Daisy's bedtime, but instead of opening this time up for an endless work session, I make a cup of tea and give myself a 2-hour maximum window. This way I stay on track, I'm more efficient, and I finish in time to wind down the evening properly and get a good night's sleep.

I enjoy communicating with the people in our Strala community around the world, and teachers and students text me all the time to chat, check in, and ask questions about their work. I could easily spend my entire day messaging back and forth, but I set boundaries here as well. I try my hardest to only check and respond to work-related chats and texts during my designated work hours. It took me some time to get over my fear of how people would react if I made them wait a day or two for a response. But it turns out that this was not the big deal I was making it out to be. If I am unable to respond for a few days, people always seem to understand and trust that I will connect when I am able to. I like to think that setting these boundaries helps others to do the same.

Afternoon Walk and Reflection Time

I try to make time for a reflective afternoon walk every day, but at minimum I make this happen three to four times a week. I'll try to take this walk after lunch, for at least 10 minutes, though I'll walk for up to an hour if I have more time. As I walk, I allow myself to daydream, to reflect on whatever is going on with me, and to pay attention to how I feel. Regardless of the season, or whether I am at home or traveling, I try to squeeze in this walk as a way to break up my workday and clear my head. I find that it's incredibly effective for making me feel refreshed and allowing me to be productive throughout the second half of my day. I highly recommend this practice for anyone who works in an office and doesn't otherwise get a lot of fresh air or exercise during the day.

Evening Meditation and Stretch

My evening meditation and stretch time is also a must. I need to check in with my body and move a bit to work out the kinks from my day. The same goes for my mind with meditation. I do this in our bedroom, usually while Mike is brushing his teeth and getting ready for bed. The scene isn't picture perfect, but that doesn't matter. I need just a few moments to get on the floor, move my body, and unwind, followed by a brief meditation to balance myself before bed. This is an easy one to fit in at the end of the day because it makes me feel so good. Really, I have no excuse not to do it! An evening stretch and meditation that I love and recommend is my Restorative Yoga Flow on page 213.

What work-life boundaries do you want to set for yourself? Grab your journal and list them. The following are the Clean Living Rules for Work-Life Balance that I recommend—you may want to adopt them all, or pick and choose from this list to suit your needs.

clean living rules for work-life balance

1. *Cultivate a hobby to restore balance.* Rather than stressing about work in your supposed free time, or living in a way that makes you feel like you are constantly plugged in and half working, carve out designed nonwork time to cultivate a new hobby. On a walk around Soho years ago with Mike, we discovered a beautiful tiny knitting shop filled with brightly colored yarn puffed up like cotton candy. We were drawn in. They were giving lessons on how to knit, and we were both so into it—it looked so fun. We ended up learning how to knit at a very basic level, and I've been making hats for friends and to donate regularly ever since. I haven't progressed past beginner level, and that's fine with me. Knitting is a hobby that is fun, relaxing, and productive. It is also meditative, so it's a great fit for my interests. It's important to find a hobby that you are actually interested in and that is fun for you. There is no need to stress out about finding a hobby. I found mine on a random walk when I least expected it. Keep your eyes and ears open as you go through your day and see where your attention is pulled.

2. *Have meaningful conversations that are not about work.* There is so much more to new people you meet, and to longtime friends and family, than what they do at work! Make it a point to engage the people you encounter in conversations that have nothing to do with what they do for a living. Talk about your favorite travel destinations, books you've read, movies you've seen, causes you are interested in, etc. This is incredibly important for cultivating balance.

3. *Schedule your meditation and movement time.* Decide on a time and schedule that is reasonable for your life, whether that is first thing in the morning, before bed, or to break up your work time, and prioritize getting in your daily movement and meditation. You need this time to listen and check in with yourself.

4. *Hang with friends who are different from you.* It's so easy to spend time with the same friends, doing the same things. This is great for comfort and our feeling of chosen family, but it's also important to spend time with friends who are different from you. Expand your comfort zone by joining groups hosted by people you admire and who are a different race or have different backgrounds and life experiences from you. If everyone you hang out with looks like you, thinks like you, and does the same things you do, that's a good clue you need to expand your circle.

5. *Read books that don't directly relate to your work.* It's so easy to exclusively consume reading materials about your field of expertise, especially if you enjoy what you do for work. It's hard not to spend all your reading time adding to your knowledge base. Allow yourself to wander into a new section in your local bookstore and see what pulls you in. Ask people who you respect and are different than you, either by their race, or background, or life experience, what they are reading, and give yourself the pleasure of escaping into and being inspired by a great book.

6. *Take vacations or staycations or daycations.* No matter how much you love what you do, taking real time away from your work is essential for your well-being. Whether you can plan a week at the beach, a few days at home, or one day to yourself, schedule time away regularly. (Holidays visiting family are wonderful but don't count in this category.)

7. *Schedule special family and friend dates.* Meet a friend for a walk and head in a direction you wouldn't normally go. Gather your family all together and cook something you've never prepared before. Take your family and friends to a local park you haven't explored. Go to a group dance class, a poetry reading, or a town hall with a friend. There is great value in discovering and learning new things with those you love.

8. *Allow yourself a goof-off day or afternoon.* We are so good at being productive, but it's important to remember that giving yourself some time to be unproductive is also useful. Follow your instinct and take a half day, an afternoon, or a full day to relax and goof off a bit when you need to. Everything you've built won't disappear if you step away for a while and have some fun. Sneak out for a movie, or take a nap or a nice, long midday bath. Hitting the refresh button occasionally is necessary for well-being.

9. *Exercise with friends or family.* Exercising with those you care about can be fun and motivating, and keeps you focused on the activity instead of worrying about work. Go for a brisk walk, jog, or side-by-side yoga session, or head to a group class. When your workout buddy is your close friend or family member, you both get healthy in the process.

10. *Regularly revisit your life goals.* It's important to revisit the big reasons you are doing all this in the first place. Do you love what you do for work, or is it a means to an end? Get real with yourself and your life goals, and stay connected to the reason you spend so much time working in the first place. Without this reflection, it's easy to stay on the hamster wheel and never be satisfied.

Remember the days when a device wasn't constantly at your fingertips, there to answer your every question with a Google search, pinging you with news updates and texts, or giving you the itch to constantly check social media? Maybe you are young enough that you have no idea what I'm talking about! If you're like me, and grew up in the eighties and nineties, you remember what it was like to truly get lost in a book, or in your imagination, without the possibility that technology would intrude. Growing up, I would actually *walk* over to a friend's house after school to see what they were up to. I might have phoned first, but usually not. When I had a question about something, there was no Google. I pulled out a giant volume of the *World Book Encyclopedia*, turned to the designated page, and found my answer in the text and glossy photos. Back then, no one could have imagined a world where instead of visiting with a friend, we might sit there texting or Snapchatting them.

Things have really changed. When I got my driver's license at sixteen, I lived in a small town called Morris in rural Illinois and my car was a Oldsmobile Delta 88 that I borrowed from my parents. I loved that car. It had an old cassette player and a soft red plush interior, and it was big enough for all my friends to pile into. When I would drive to school or to my after-school job or to dance class, my parents would remind me to take our *portable phone* with me. That's right, this was 1997, and in those days a portable phone came with a giant black case that resembled carry-on luggage. I was only to use the car phone in an absolute emergency, like if the car got stuck in a ditch and no one would stop to help me. I never actually made a call on that phone because of how much I thought it would cost my parents. And thankfully, I never had an emergency that would have called for me to use it. Sometimes I think back on the security that never-used car phone provided. I breathed easier knowing that if something happened, I could pick it up and call for help.

Technology today seems to have the opposite effect. It makes us feel insecure and anxious. Instead of making our lives easier, it just makes us busier. The options and possibilities are limitless, and this has the effect of making us unfocused, stressed, and addicted to constantly checking our phones for an update, for that little dopamine reward we get when someone likes our new Instagram post. Technology has completely changed the way we think about ourselves and relate to the world, and it is a huge challenge to have a healthy relationship with our devices. But it is possible. We just have to tap into what we already know and have known all along: the universe is not contained in your phone! There is a big world out there, so go outside, interact with other people and with nature, and have fun.

Don't Be Tied to Your Devices

We can change our habits when it comes to technology, but first we must have the desire to change. How do you want to feel after interacting with your phone, your computer, and your other devices? How do you want these devices to serve you? You guessed it—write those things down! Here are some examples:

- I want to feel like my use of technology supports my creativity, rather than diminishing it.

- I want to feel connected to my friends and inspired by those I follow, not jealous or drained by seeing so much content.

- I want to feel informed and energized by what's going on in the world, not obsessed with or overwhelmed by constant news updates and everyone's opinions and commentary.

- I want to feel inspired professionally and continue my education to improve my skills.

CLEAN MIND DIGITAL DETOX

Technology habits in conflict with your goals? Adjust your screen time and device use around the way you want to feel. The average American checks their phone eighty times a day. That's an alarming statistic. Living your life is not the same as *sharing* every moment of your life. Here are a few digital detox practices to institute throughout your Mental Cleanse week, to help you take back control and regain your creativity, your peace of mind, and your life.

Establish a Tech-Free Morning Routine

A healthy morning routine is essential for setting the tone for the rest of your entire day. I used to sleep with my phone charging on my nightstand, and it would be the first thing I reached for when I opened my eyes in the morning (or in the middle of the night, when I couldn't sleep!). This was not a healthy habit! Today, my tech-free morning routine involves sleeping *without* my phone—I charge it in a separate room, and you should do the same. Upon waking, before I even get out of bed, I do my Clean Mind breathing practice, mentioned at the start of this chapter. Then I practice 10 minutes of movement and meditation, usually before making breakfast for everyone. Either Mike or I will get Daisy out of bed and ready for breakfast. We don't have a rigid schedule and we take turns depending on what's going on that day. We eat breakfast together and hang out for a bit before Mike takes Daisy to school and I start my workday. This is when I first pick up my phone for the day.

Whatever the schedule of your morning is, it's a classic no-no to pick up your phone first thing. Keep your phone out of your bedroom. You can't reach for what isn't there. It might be a massive challenge to overcome the addiction of reaching for your phone first thing in the morning. Go easy on yourself and keep trying. Plan a brief morning routine that is just for you and know that everything inside your phone will still be there when you decide to pick it up.

Many of us keep a phone in the bedroom at night because we use it as an alarm. Is this really an excuse? Shift this needless habit by investing in a simple digital or analog clock for your nightstand. It might seem more convenient to use your phone, but it's terrible for your overall well-being. Make your bedroom a sanctuary for rest and sleep and make your morning routine sacred. A good night's sleep and a mindful morning routine will set the tone for your entire day.

Set Boundaries Around Social Media, News, and TV Consumption

Your phone now has settings that track your daily and weekly usage, and will alert you when you've been using it for a certain length of time. Many apps have this function as well. Get in the habit of tracking your screen time on your phone. Once you start paying attention, the amount of time you are spending on your phone or on particular apps might surprise you. I set my Instagram alert to go off after 30 minutes of use, and this is my limit for the day. I'll admit that the first time I did this, the alert went off very early in the day! I was shocked how much time I was spending on Instagram. I use the app to communicate with my yoga community, but I've decided that for me, 30 minutes is enough. Once I set this limit and started sticking to it, I realized that I'd been telling myself I was spending the time for productive purposes when really I was mindlessly scrolling.

With the news, it's of course important to stay informed. But with the relentless pace of the news cycle these days, combined with constant coverage of events large and small, and our seemingly limitless access to news via online sources, print, and TV, it's easy for obsessive, unhealthy behavior to form. During this detox period, limit yourself to one designated time of day when you will check the news, for a maximum of one hour, whether that's reading the news online, watching a TV news program, or reading the physical newspaper (assuming that anyone out there does that anymore!).

Leave Your Phone at Home

This doesn't have to be for the entire day, and it may not be practical for you on a workday. Start small, on the weekend, by leaving your phone at home while you go for a short walk, out to dinner, or to an event. The idea behind this exercise is to practice being present and at peace with your thoughts, whether you are out alone or with another person, and the more you do it, the easier it will get. It sounds radical, I know. But as much as you can during this detox period, try using your phone exclusively as the emergency contact device that it is.

Stop Scrolling—and Carry a Book!

Mindless scrolling during everyday activities like commuting on public transportation, and waiting in line at the store has become so common—we barely notice we are doing it. Many of us even do this while walking down city streets, which is just plain dangerous. Stop scrolling! This practice is pointless, and it drains your mental energy. Instead, carry a book with you and read during your commute or while waiting in line. During an elevator ride, take a few breaths and a moment of silence to yourself, or say hello to the person next to you! These shifts will improve your well-being and your mental state considerably.

Screen Time and Kids

As the mother of a three-year-old, I always have this issue at the top of my mind. When it comes to little ones, we are all so concerned about the damage that new technology is potentially causing. The trouble is, there's still not a ton of conclusive research in this area, because technology is constantly changing and it's all so new. But one thing we can be certain of is that our kids are always watching what we are doing. If you are constantly on your laptop or checking your phone, you are teaching your kids that your device is the center of your world. Repairing your habits and setting limits for yourself when it comes to technology is essential before you can even begin to teach your kids about what is appropriate and important.

Here are a few good ground rules when it comes to little ones and screen time.

Watch Together

There are a couple of great educational kids' shows that Mike and I allow Daisy to watch, but our rule is that we watch them with her. There is a big difference between watching a show with your child and giving your child an iPhone or tablet or putting them in front of the TV to keep them busy. Watching together allows you to talk about the show, sing the songs together, and of course snuggle. Using a phone or a tablet is an isolating act, so as much as possible, try to avoid handing your child a device to keep them busy. We all want attention from people, and giving our attention to our children is the best we can offer. It's important not to be too rigid when it comes to kids and tech, but at the same time, we must realize that if tech is addictive and depleting for adults, it must have a similar effect on children.

Offer Fun Screen-Free Alternatives

Come up with a list of fun, old-fashioned, screen-free activities that you and your kids already do together or could start doing together. Write these down and keep the list pinned to your fridge or bulletin board so that it's at the ready on weekends or on a rainy day. Our favorite no-tech indoor activities include baking cookies, making smoothies, playing catch and kick with a balloon, playing hide-and-seek, popping bubble wrap, and reading picture books. We also take any opportunity we can get to be outside, and our favorite outdoor activities are drawing with sidewalk chalk, going for a walk in our neighborhood, going to the playground or park, or kicking a ball around the yard. Devise your own lists based on your kids' ages, activities levels, and what your family loves to do!

Check Your Own Habits

Kids can sense when you are distracted, even if you are across the room. When you are with little ones, be extra mindful of your technology use. Of course, sometimes you need to make a call or answer an email, but do your best to avoid mindlessly scrolling when you are with your kids. And when you do have to use your phone or device, explain what you are doing. For example, tell them, "I am doing some work right now, but as soon as I finish, we can play." Mike and I try to do this as much as possible, and now, when Daisy sees one of us on our phone, she understands what is going on; she'll say, "Dada is working," and run to play with me, or the other way around. We want her to know that these devices are for specific purposes and are not the most important things in our lives.

NOURISHING RELATIONSHIPS

The final step in your Mental Cleanse is devoted to the important relationships in your life with the people you see on a daily basis—your family members, your friends, and your coworkers. Any relationship in your life, whether it is with a loved one or a colleague, needs to be grounded in communication and trust to succeed. These relationships begin with you, and doing the inner work needed to connect with those around you.

My favorite way to think about successful relationships begins with this simple truth: our relationships with others reflect the relationships we are having with ourselves. When our inner ecosystems are swirling with anxiety and stress, it is difficult, if not impossible, to connect with those around us. Whether we are aware of it or not, we are all leaders. We lead with the energy we put out into the world, and that energy is contagious. It affects everyone we encounter. When we are in touch with our best selves, conversations with strangers happen spontaneously and are full of joy and hope. Work interactions are full of purpose and passion. Family life is fun and rejuvenating. By contrast, when we are feeling stuck and disconnected from ourselves, or are tense, anxious, or depressed, this will manifest in our relationships with other people. These interactions will become dark and heavy, or laden with tension and anxiety.

Dealing with Difficult People

Change begins with you. You may be living in a reactive mode, blaming the difficult people around you and absorbing their negative energy. But guess what? You have the power to change the way you relate to the people in your life. You can shift the energy in your relationships by doing the inner work to prepare for these encounters. Ground yourself, project confidence and positive energy, and decide that *you* will set the tone, rather than reacting—and reacting negatively—to difficult, seemingly toxic people in your life.

I know how challenging this can be, believe me. I have been there. Shifting the tone in a dysfunctional relationship does not mean that the difficult people around you will suddenly be easy to get along with. But you can change the way you show up to these encounters, and the way you react to them. Begin by finding balance and harmony within. That deep connection with yourself will extend to your connections with others.

Your Relationship with *You*

Staying connected with your inner self takes fierce dedication and commitment. You need to carve out time in your schedule, on a regular basis, to check in with yourself, and to reflect on your goals and what you want to achieve in your life. This begins with a morning routine that makes you feel great and sets the stage for the rest of your day. And it continues with finding moments throughout your day to check in with your breath and your thoughts. Maintaining this connection with yourself is essential to having healthy relationships with others. Self-care isn't selfish. It is critical to bringing your best to every situation.

When you are living your life at warp speed, it is inevitable that you are going to crash into the people around you and wreak havoc. By contrast, when we take the time to reflect on our relationship with ourselves, this benefits the people around us, too. By building alone time and reflection into your daily routine, each interaction you have becomes more graceful and meaningful.

The next time you have a free moment and are tempted to reach for a distraction—whether that means checking social media or answering a stray email—see if you can take the time to be with yourself instead. It's almost unheard of to see someone sitting alone in a coffee shop with just their thoughts, not scrolling through their phone. Let's make quality time with ourselves a more common occurrence! During this reflection time, set an intention for how you would like your relationships to feel. Whether you are looking for more creativity, openness, support, or meaning, setting an intention is like clearing a path toward what you want. It's a reminder to be more mindful so as to foster better connections.

These are my favorite practices for reconnecting with myself in order to make space for good relationships with others.

Alone Time

Make a point to have a date with yourself once a week. During this time, commit to really sitting with your thoughts. Go to a coffee shop, or out to lunch or dinner, and leave your phone at home. Be brave! If going out alone makes you self-conscious, take comfort in knowing 99 percent of the time no one is paying attention to what you are doing. Everyone is absorbed in their own thoughts and worlds. You're good. While you are out on your solo date, pay attention to your breath, and notice how you feel. Are you tempted to distract yourself from your thoughts in some way? Are you uncomfortable without your phone? Notice these things as they come up and keep breathing deeply.

Inspiration Walks

Walks are a great way to reconnect with yourself and tap into your creativity and inspiration. Particularly if you are feeling stuck or in a rut, changing your environment, boosting your blood flow, and breathing some fresh air by going for a walk can do wonders. As I mentioned on page 40, I like to take a reflective afternoon walk every day if I can, but three or four times a week at minimum. These walks don't just have to happen in the afternoon. I'll go out for an inspiration walk any time I'm feeling like I need a fresh perspective, including before I teach a yoga retreat or a training session, or before and after important meetings to get the ideas flowing and allow myself to be more open to feedback. Don't wait until you hit a roadblock to set off on an inspiration walk. Make these part of your practice, and incorporate a reflective, head-clearing walk into your routine once a week for at least 30 minutes.

Reflective Journaling

We all know that journaling can be cathartic, but it is also a practice that benefits your relationships. Give yourself a writing assignment: Write an entry in your journal on past and present relationships in your life that are or have been negative and positive, and write about the kinds of relationships you want to build in the future. Focus on what you can control—you—rather than on the other people in these relationships. In past relationships, how could you have handled things differently? How could you have established healthier boundaries, been of more service, or been more present and engaged? Do you notice patterns in your life with the way you feel about yourself and the kinds of relationships you are having? If you aren't happy with these patterns, what can you do to make a change? Take the time to examine relationships with friends, family, romantic partners, mentors, coworkers, and any future relationships you would like to have.

"be moved" meditation practice

We can't have healthy relationships without give and take, and what I call being "moveable" is essential to any good relationship. This means that we need to be open to our friends, partners, and family members so that we allow ourselves to be moved by their thoughts, feelings, and needs. We want these people to remain moveable toward us in turn. Being moveable is the opposite of remaining rigid and stuck in our ways. The trees are moveable in the wind. Can you imagine how silly it would be if a tree resisted the breeze? We can practice this way of being with a simple meditation.

1. Sit comfortably. Relax your body and let yourself settle in with yourself. Close your eyes.

2. Take a full, deep inhale, followed by a full, deep exhale. Continue breathing deeply, inhaling and exhaling, and pay attention to the way your breath allows your body to expand and relaxes you.

3. Allow your body to move slowly in any direction that feels good to you, in response to your breath. If you find a place that feels tight, stay there for a few deep breaths. Pay attention to whether anything opens up or changes as you breathe. Continue to explore and move with your breath for a few moments. Breathing deeply will show you where your body is asking for attention, allow your body to release

tension, and give you information about what is going on with you emotionally.

4. When you are ready, return to center and stillness. In this stillness, notice your body continuing to lift and lower very gently with your breath. This isn't a big, visible movement, but you will notice a soft lifting and lowering, like a wave. This is you being moveable. Notice how you feel.

Practice Active Listening

One of the best things we can do to improve our relationships is get better at listening. Too often we are simply waiting for our turn to talk or talking over another person. The next time you're in a conversation with someone, practice active listening. Rather than waiting for your chance to respond, *really listen.* Observe their body language, and the energy they are giving off, in addition to what they are saying to you. As you actively listen, be sure to keep breathing, especially if the conversation is getting heated or you don't like what the other person is saying. Wait for the other person to finish, and take your time in responding. Practice being direct and thoughtful with your response.

Keep in mind that we also get into the habit of using filler words such as "like," "um," and "you know," and that these take away from the power of what we are trying to communicate. Take your time when you respond. Speak slowly and clearly. When the impulse to use filler words comes up, take a breath and a true pause. Active listening is a profound practice that will improve your relationships, your ability to communicate, and your confidence the more you do it.

Nourishing the Positive Relationships in Your Life

Let's not forget that it's also important to make space and time to nourish the relationships in your life that are going well, and not to take these relationships for granted. Whether the relationship in question is with your partner, a close friend, a family member, or a favorite coworker, the more care you put into connecting with these special people, the more happiness, joy, and comfort you'll receive. It's so easy to take the people close to us for granted. They are always around. They will show up when you need a shoulder to cry on or a date to an event. Make it a priority to spend quality time with these people outside your usual interactions.

One great way of doing this is to cook a special meal together, for no reason other than to show this person how much you value spending time with them. Another fun way is to have a coloring party with friends. I used to do this back when I was in dance conservatory. I would invite people over to my dorm room for coloring parties, and we would relax and unwind together with a bunch of coloring books and crayons and a bottle of wine. At the end of the evening, we'd trade our finished "artwork" with each other, and my walls ended up plastered with colorful, quirky art that brought me so much joy.

People Who Are Living It Right

In this section, I'd like to introduce you to some people I admire who are living the Clean Mind practices and principles outlined in this chapter. Take a cue from the way these awesome folks are living as you embark on your mental reset! (Note: All interviews featured in this book were conducted prior to the pandemic, before social distancing orders were implemented.)

COURTNEY NICHOLS GOULD
Founder of SmartyPants Vitamins, on Boundaries, Family Time, and Oat Milk Lattes

Courtney Nichols Gould is a former tech start-up executive who was COO of Clear, the airport security fast pass, before starting her company, SmartyPants Vitamins. She founded SmartyPants with Gordon, an old acquaintance who would end up becoming her husband. Courtney and Gordon fell in love while building the company, got married, and now they live in Venice Beach, California, with Gordon's two children, Kylan, 17, and Oliver, 15.

Courtney manages to do the seemingly impossible, remaining balanced personally and professionally while running a company with her husband and juggling a busy life with two stepchildren. Courtney is incredibly passionate, and she brings a rare kind of integrity to her work. In 2012, there was a global shortage of natural vitamin E, a common ingredient in SmartyPants Vitamins. The company had 48 hours to decide between being sold out for 6 months or using synthetic vitamin E in their product. The synthetic version isn't dangerous, but the body doesn't absorb it as well as natural vitamin E. Courtney chose to ask her consumers via email what they preferred. The company communicated the situation clearly, and they received consistent responses from their customers saying they understood the situation and asking SmartyPants to please continue making the vitamins with the synthetic vitamin until the natural version was available again. Because of her transparency with her customers, what could have been a crisis turned into a way to build brand trust, and her revenue grew by 170 percent that year. She brings this same openness and integrity to her personal life.

How do you set boundaries around technology with your kids?

We have a couple of firm rules in our house. I tell my kids, no cell phones until age 13, screen time ends 45 minutes before bed, and no phones at the table ever—that includes their parents! That last one is my favorite. I love never having my phone at a meal, whether with family or friends, and I think the kids appreciate the designated break. Beyond these ground rules, my husband and I try to teach the kids discernment when it comes to technology use. Because their judgment is what will serve them best in the long run!

What activities do you do to connect as a family?

Our favorites ways to connect are having dinner together, spending time together in nature, and visiting new places like art museums together. And there's no shame in lounging around watching a movie together after a long, activity-filled day—it's a good way to sneak in hugs and kisses with the kids as they get older! The kids and I also like to listen to podcasts together on the drive to school. This is a great way to get them talking and to get a sense of what they are thinking and the way their minds work!

How do you connect with your creative side?

My favorite way to reconnect with my creativity is to be silent— hiking with our dogs at dawn is very good for this—or else being with a group of friends and talking out ideas over a delicious meal. Some of the best ideas come from smart people operating outside their area of expertise. I also love going to conferences to hear about new brilliant ideas related to random topics.

What is your morning routine?

I meditate for 20 minutes, preferably in the bubble chair in my daughter's room. Then I drink hot water with lemon and head out to walk the dogs for a good sweat. I stop off at Cha Cha Matcha for an oat milk latte (seriously heaven, and that place is my new obsession). I head home to get ready and then I'm off to whatever my day holds. This is my morning routine for a calm and open mind, and a happy body and soul. I feel the difference when my day doesn't begin with this routine.

SHELAH BERGBOWER

Farmer, on Art, Community, and Lessons from the Family Farm

My cousin Shelah runs a farm in Newton, Illinois, on which several members of my extended family work. The farm was started by our great-grandfather on my mother's side, with its main barns located up a gravel road behind our grandmother's home. I grew up hearing stories about my mom cooking large dinners for her four brothers, who all worked on the farm from a young age. Everyone pitched in and everyone worked hard. Shelah, of the next generation, also grew up driving a tractor and working the fields as a kid, alongside her dad and her brothers, Todd and Tony. Tony left for the big city of St. Louis after college, but Todd and Shelah can be found in the fields or taking care of the farm equipment most days. Shelah is married to a non-farmer named Chad. They have two children, Alex, 15, and Ethan, 20.

Shelah and I have been deeply connected since we were kids, when we would stay up all night drinking tea, pretending we were big bosses, and working on art projects together. I eventually began dreaming of city life, but Shelah has always loved horses, wide-open spaces, and the rhythms of the country. She is constantly engaged in some sort of fun project with her kids or busy volunteering in her community. Shelah's creative projects have included renovating an old farmhouse that her family now lives in and building a gorgeous modern barn, complete with horse stables and gardens. In many ways, our lives couldn't have gone in two more different directions, but we have some major common threads, which is why I love comparing notes on the ways we find balance.

How do you create an environment of calm for yourself and your family in the midst of a hectic, stressful farm life?

The key is to have a plan. I try to plan things out so that all the little things in our daily routine are squared away before the day even begins. If we can avoid a morning crisis like running out of toothpaste, for example, that's a win. I also try to prepare family meals in advance and stash them in the freezer, so that there is something easy we can pop in the oven for dinner at the end of a long day.

How do you find creative inspiration in everyday life?

I have been a farmer all my life, and farming is hard work! I think it's important to balance that out by nurturing your creative side. In our small, rural community there aren't many natural opportunities for kids to express themselves creatively, so I started leading art workshops throughout the year to fix that. If ever you are looking for inspiration, go talk to some kids! They are so open to new ideas, and they're not limited by the concepts that seem to fence us in as adults. Like I tell my kids in art class, only you can decide when your project is done and only you can call it good. What other people think doesn't matter. What matters is what makes you happy.

Who has been a source of inspiration to you?

Our grandma! She used to say to me, "I can't die today, I have too many things that need to get done tomorrow." As a kid, I remember thinking, "What does she have to do? Grandmas don't do anything." When I look back, I realize how busy she was, making cookies for me to take to school to share with friends, or making stuffed animals and dolls to give as gifts. I see now that she spent her time investing in the lives of others. That is the greatest purpose anyone can have in life, I believe.

Do you have a daily ritual for staying centered?

My daily routine varies, depending on the season. In the summer, there's nothing quite like starting the day on the porch with a cup of tea and my dog, watching the sun rise, the hummingbirds zooming by, and the horses on our farm sunning themselves. This brings me a sense of peace. Winter means craft time: crocheting, baking, and painting all bring me to my quiet, centered place.

2

hit the reset:

spiritual detox

Resting in Awareness we transform the "stuff" of our lives.
—Ram Dass

At a certain point in our lives, many of us begin to crave deeper meaning and purpose. We ask ourselves questions like, "Am I doing what I was put on this earth to do?" or "Am I just going through the motions?" We may call this questioning a midlife crisis or a quarter-life crisis, depending on our life stage. I call this moment a "crisis of spirit." The search for deeper meaning and purpose, against the backdrop of our busy lives, can be a source of stress and angst. But I believe that each of us is born with a true sense of our greater purpose. We may lose track of it as life progresses and becomes more complicated. We may get closer to it and drift away again at different times in our lives, influenced by external circumstances and the expectations of others. But we can always return to it.

The goal of Week 2 of your *Clean Mind, Clean Body* journey is to reconnect to your spiritual purpose, or possibly to find it for the first time. In the day-to-day of our busy lives, it can be challenging to stay connected to a greater sense of purpose. Often we leave our spiritual lives and finding a sense of purpose for last, thinking that nurturing this side of ourselves is a luxury we rarely have time for. Or else the search to reconnect with this purpose begins with something big and dramatic—a life event that serves as a wake-up call or a rock-bottom moment. But we don't have to wait for something dramatic to occur to get on the spiritual path.

My goal for you during this week is to recognize that cultivating your spiritual side should be part of your daily practice. I want you to feel aligned with a greater sense of purpose in all that you do throughout the course of your day. And ultimately, I want this purpose to be what leads, guides, pulls, and carries you through life, during both good and challenging times. This chapter is about rediscovering, in the most fundamental way, what it means to be uniquely, wonderfully you.

We are all spiritual creatures, even if we don't fully realize it. Try thinking back to a time as a kid when you felt completely yourself, relaxed and comfortable, unconcerned with the expectations of others, and inspired. Maybe it was when you were doing something that you loved, like a favorite childhood hobby. Maybe it was a simple moment, but one where you felt really alive, like lying in your backyard in the grass and staring up at the sky. I remember a moment like this, when I was around seven years old. I was sitting in the woods behind my house and I was suddenly hit with a profound understanding of who I was and my connection to the vast universe that I was a part of. I remember completely losing track of time, and my physical senses taking over, sounds around me becoming clearer, and colors brighter. I got this message from the universe that I had been put on earth to help others, to serve in some way, and I remember feeling excited that my life was so full of potential in that moment.

I know this story may sound a little out there, particularly the idea that this happened to me as a seven-year-old. But the truth is that we are all capable of receiving these kinds of messages from the universe about our purpose, if we are willing to be open and listen for them. I believe that that moment, at age seven, was ultimately what led me to my calling as a yoga teacher—even if I lost my way and veered off this path occasionally. My decision to change my life, slow down, and reprioritize, which I talked about in the previous chapter, was what led me to rediscover this path and my purpose.

Reconnecting with our spiritual side as adults can be a profound and comforting experience. I'd compare it to opening a dresser drawer, rediscovering a favorite, perfectly worn-in sweater, and putting it on—the feeling is at once new and invigorating, and familiar. But we make this process of reconnecting with our spirituality more difficult than it should be. Often, we ignore our spirit until a painful or unpleasant experience serves as a wake-up call, bringing us back to what is truly important in life. It's easy to go through life on autopilot, ignoring what is not serving us, until something stops us in our tracks. Whether this wake-up call arrives in the form of burnout, illness, or tragedy, it jolts us into action and forces us to change. For some of us, multiple wake-up calls are needed. Even after one of these shocks to the system sets us off in search of something better, the spark of change fades. Soon enough we're back in a rut. We get stuck living this way because it is more comfortable to do what's familiar, even if it isn't working.

My friend Stu was an example of someone who lived this way, alternating between unhealthy lifestyle choices that weren't serving him and spiritually "awake" phases in his life when he felt a deep connection to his purpose. Stu was a great guy with a huge heart, and was naturally outgoing, a people person. During these awake phases, he was full of energy, seeking healthy ways to nourish himself and making positive connections with those around him. Naturally built like a big brown bear, as broad shouldered as he was tall, Stu was also someone who took some risks with his health.

His weight fluctuated dramatically depending on how well he was taking care of himself, and whether he was stressed out and eating poorly or on a yoga kick. In his early forties, Stu was diagnosed with cancer.

I visited Stu in the hospital and then at home during his first round of cancer treatments. I cooked some of my favorite healthy meals for him and we spent time joking and goofing off and doing yoga together. Stu went through phases where he committed to changing his lifestyle, vowing to do all he could to fight the cancer by dialing down his stress, eating more plant-based and fewer processed foods, and practicing yoga more regularly. But when I visited Stu in the hospital during his second round of treatments, he wasn't as motivated to stay on the path, and he seemed disconnected and defensive when I asked him what he was doing to stay healthy. He was still happy to have my company, however, joking that he couldn't wait to get out of the hospital so he could eat some fast food—that was so Stu. Stu was dying, and we both knew there wasn't a magic soup that would fix this.

In Stu's case, it would be unfair to say that healthier habits would have prevented him from getting cancer or kept him alive once he got his cancer diagnosis. It's important to understand that health is multifactorial, a combination of lifestyle choices and genetics, and that even when we make healthy choices, our bodies are still vulnerable to illness. The big lesson I learned from Stu was not so much about lifestyle choices, but about spiritual presence. When Stu was in his healthy phases, he was fully alive, awake, and spiritually connected. Healthy habits are a part of that, but they're not the endpoint. When we spend our time obsessing over healthy lifestyle choices, we're missing the bigger picture. The true goal is to maintain our health so that we can live a life we love and do the things that fulfill us and bring us joy. Stu's story reminds us that life is a beautiful gift and that we never know how long we will be here to enjoy it.

I often wonder if it was exhausting for Stu to cycle between his destructive phases and his spiritually awake phases. I wonder how many chances each of us is given to stray from our purpose and then return to it. I cherish the memories I have of Stu and the joy we shared. Thinking of him reminds me not to lose that connection to my purpose and, when I notice that I'm drifting, to come back.

How often do you catch yourself thinking, "I'll be happier, or I'll take better care of my health, when this happens or that happens"? Thinking this way, especially when it comes to health and lifestyle choices, is a trap. It's living according to a deferred life plan. If you want to live with a true sense of connection and well-being, you need to start changing your life now. A friend of mine spent a lot of time with spiritual teacher Ram Dass in his last years, and told me that when Dass passed away, he left with "no gas in the tank," meaning he had given his all. I believe that we should all try to live this way, staying connected to our purpose, loving and enjoying our lives and each other while we are here, and leaving with no gas left in the tank.

Finding Your Spiritual Flow

Flow state, also known as "being in the zone," is a mental state in which a person performing an activity is fully immersed, and experiences a feeling of energized focus, full involvement, and enjoyment of the activity. Psychologist Mihály Csíkszentmihályi coined the term "flow" in 1975, and it became a leading principle of the positive psychology movement. "Flow" more recently has been used across a variety of fields, but the concept has existed for thousands of years under other names in Eastern religions such as Hinduism, Buddhism, Taoism, and Sufism, and is expressed in these traditions through meditation, prayer, and the healing and martial arts.

One benefit of the flow state that can be achieved through meditation is what is referred to as the "relaxation response." This term was coined by Dr. Herbert Benson, a Harvard physician, and is discussed in his book of the same name. Benson defines the relaxation response as a person's ability to encourage their body to release chemicals and brain signals that make their muscles and organs slow down and increase blood flow to the brain. In the 1960s and '70s, Benson conducted studies that showed meditation promotes better health, especially in individuals with hypertension, lowering stress levels, increasing well-being, and even reducing blood pressure and resting heart rate.

The relaxation response is essentially the opposite of the fight-or-flight stress response, and it brings the body back to a place of healing and repair. The more time we can spend in a state of relaxation response and flow, the healthier and more spiritually connected we become. Our culture tends to celebrate the quick fix rather than the kind of relaxation and slowing down that accompanies physical practices with a spiritual component like yoga and meditation. For most of us, moving to an ashram just isn't practical, but we can remember that we achieve the benefits of these spiritual practices when we slow down and tune in to ourselves, rather than tuning out.

Flow lives inside us, waiting to be activated through these practices. We've all experienced it at one time or another, and it's like muscle memory—we always have access to it. I used to lead Deepak Chopra and his wife, Rita, in morning yoga practice at their home, and I loved the way Deepak would describe the flow state activated by yoga. After we finished a session, he would often say that during our practice we had been "nonlocal," meaning that we'd had the experience of being there doing yoga, but also of being present with a bigger sense of awareness. In flow state, you're there, but you also somehow feel like you're everywhere.

I like to do a little experiment when I lead Strala Teacher Trainings. I'll lead my students in a short yoga sequence, and I'll make the deliberate choice to do so without being fully present. I'll call out the poses and say all the right things, but the connection to myself is missing. After the exercise, I bring everyone together and ask for feedback. It's easy to see before everyone starts talking that the sequence felt awkward. Students report wanting the exercise to be over; feeling less confident and off-balance, causing them to push through poses and stumble; and feeling disconnected from themselves during the sequence. Then I lead the sequence again, this time centering myself and connecting my body and breath, which brings me into the moment. I feel "in flow" with the class, like we are breathing together, even though I am the leader. There is an enjoyable dance happening, instead of an authority figure giving instructions to a disempowered group blindly following and not at all listening to their inner guide. We come together again for a discussion, and the feedback is always dramatically different this time around. People report feeling "in flow," being able to do so much more physically, and wanting the exercise to continue when I call for it to end.

I do this exercise in my trainings to demonstrate that flow state is always there, but it's easy to miss if we're not fully present. The magic of yoga isn't about the sequence, it's about the connection. If you are leading yoga or simply in a conversation with another person, your connection to yourself drives the feeling of that interaction. Your connection to yourself either turns flow state on and makes room for something positive to happen, or it shuts flow state off and limits possibilities.

SPIRITUAL GOAL SETTING

When it comes to goal setting for your Spiritual Detox, the first thing to keep in mind is that you are *already* spiritual, even if you've temporarily lost touch with your spiritual side. Reconnecting with your spirituality isn't about decorating your home with crystals or meditating to make up for the fact that you are acting like a stressed-out jerk most of the time. True spirituality lies in remembering who you are at your very core. It is about the way you treat yourself, and those around you, on an average day. Our actions toward ourselves and toward each other on a daily basis are our true spiritual practices. And what we practice on a daily basis grows stronger, bringing us closer to or pushing us farther away from our spiritual nature.

As you work toward your spiritual goals, keep in mind that being spiritually connected isn't about walking around decked out in mala beads and wishing everyone blessings as you go through your day. It's about living strongly connected to your purpose, feeling wide awake and grateful to be alive, and having the ability to use your time and energy to live life to the fullest of your potential. Your spirituality should look and feel like you. This is a change that happens internally, like a glow that lights you from the inside out.

Like the Mental Detox in the previous chapter, the Spiritual Detox portion of our journey is also a one-week process. The goal is to dive in fully and build on the Mental Detox practices from the previous week. The areas of focus for our Spiritual Detox week are:

- *Meditation:* We'll remove spiritual blockages, create a daily meditation practice, and make it last.

- *Slowing Down:* We'll focus on setting a more aware and tuned-in pace of life, aligning with nature, and gaining a reflective practice.

- *Living with Intention:* We'll create mindful moments and movements out of everyday tasks and detoxing from negative patterns of thought.

clean mind, clean body

SAMPLE DAILY ROUTINES

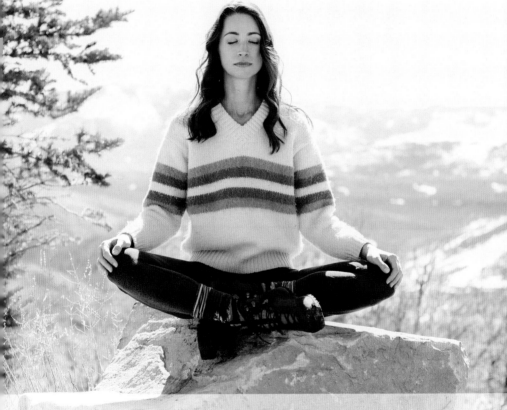

Here are some examples of how your days might look during the 28-day detox period of your *Clean Mind, Clean Body* journey. These sample daily routines are intended to guide and inspire you, and they are meant to be flexible. Feel free to change it up to keep things interesting, and to add and subtract, depending on your schedule and energy levels throughout each week!

mental detox

8 AM	Morning Yoga Stretch
9 AM	Meditation for a Healing Space
10 AM	Cleaning with Kids
12 PM	Cultivate a Hobby to Restore Balance
2 PM	Afternoon Walk and Reflection Time
5 PM	Nourish Positive Relationships
6 PM	Reflective Journaling
8 PM	Evening Meditation and Stretch

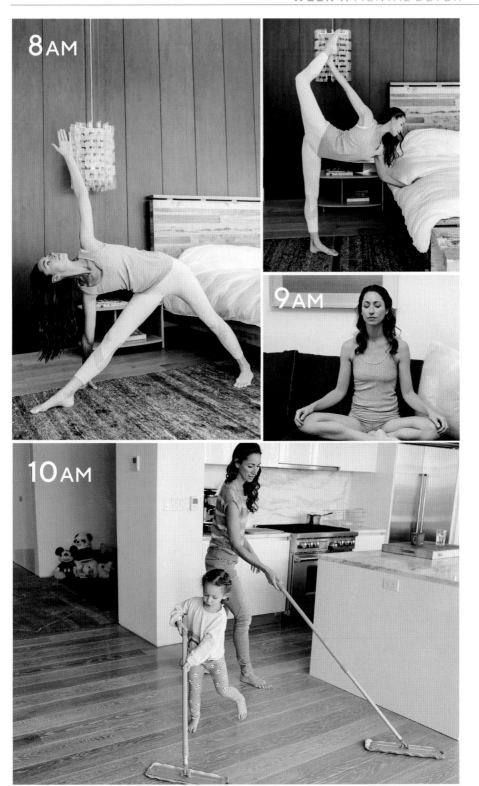

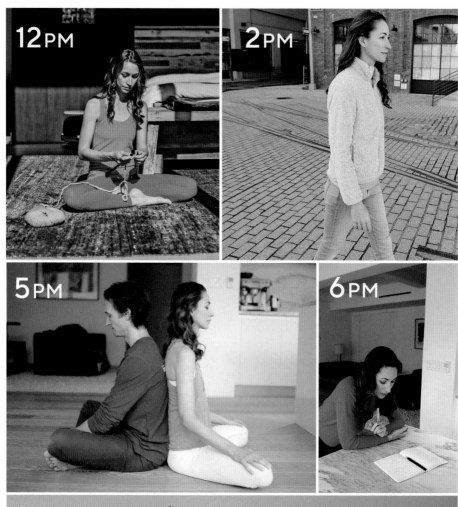

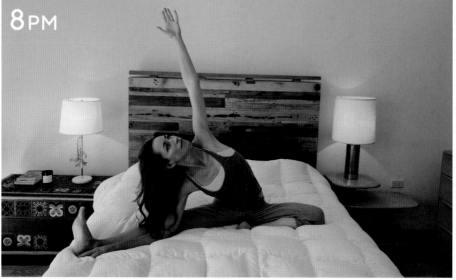

spiritual detox

8 AM	Morning Meditation
10 AM	Self-Shiatsu
12 PM	Pleasure Reading
2 PM	Nature Walk
4 PM	Afternoon Meditation
6 PM	Reflective Journaling

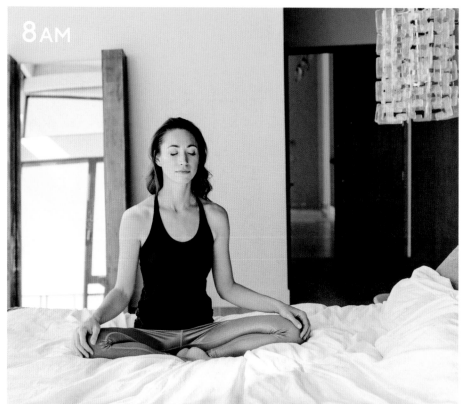

8 AM

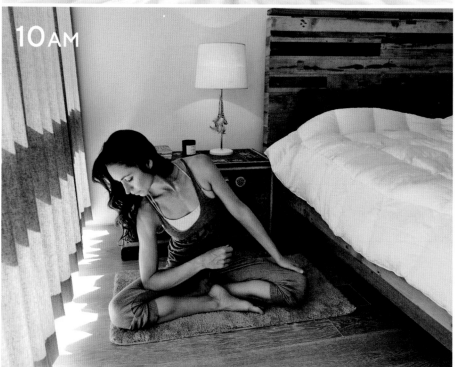

10 AM

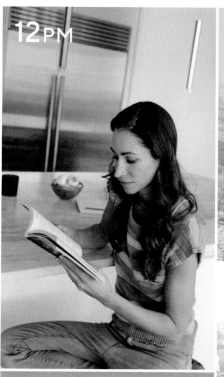

12PM

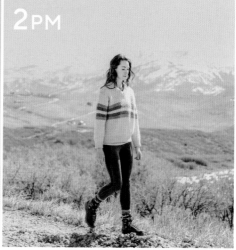

2PM

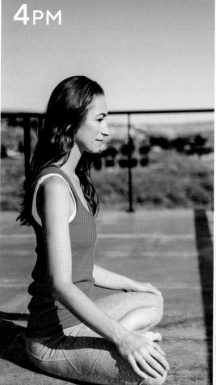

4PM

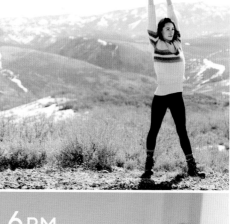

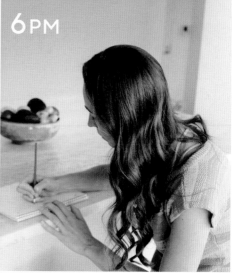

6PM

Week 3

change the way you eat

---

8 AM Morning Meditation and Yoga Stretch

10 AM Turmeric Latte

12 PM Everyday Kitchari

2 PM Pick Up Fresh Produce at Your Local Farmers' Market

4 PM Afternoon Meditation

6 PM Reflective Journaling

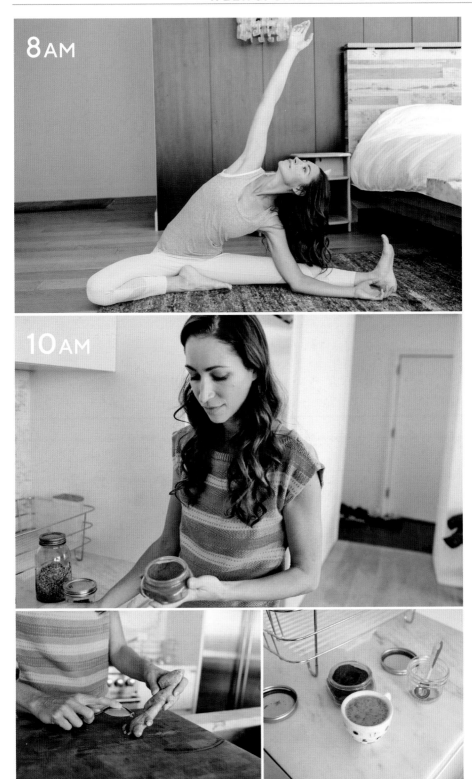

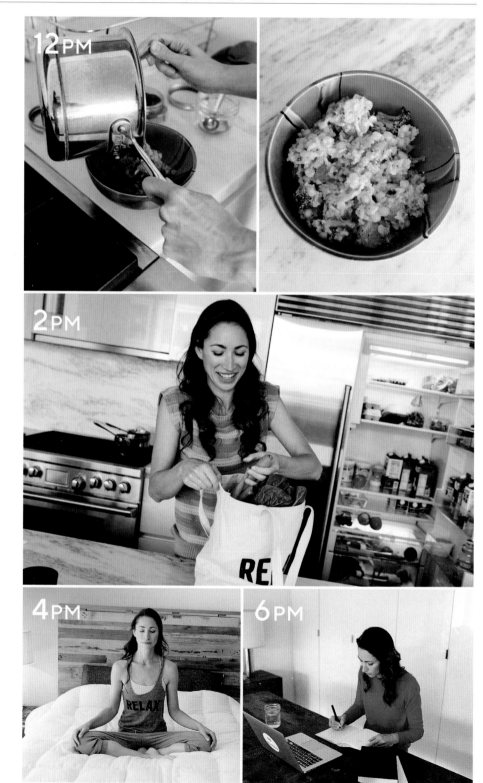

change the way you move

8 AM Tai Chi Wake and Shake

10 AM Exercises for the Office

5:30 PM *Seasonal Movement:* Spring Rebirth Yoga Routine

6:30 PM Exercises While Cooking:

Blender Balancing Act

Wait and Bake

8:30 PM Evening Yoga Wind-Down

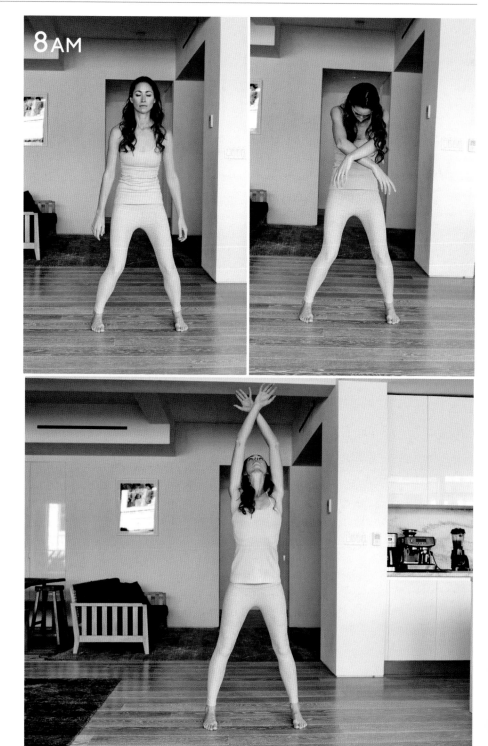

8AM

tai-chi wake and shake

exercises for the office

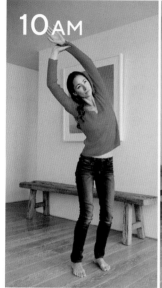
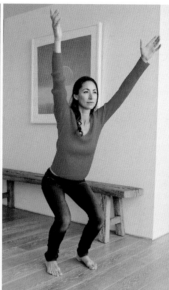
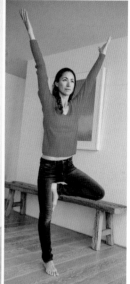

10AM

side stretch   squats   tree pose

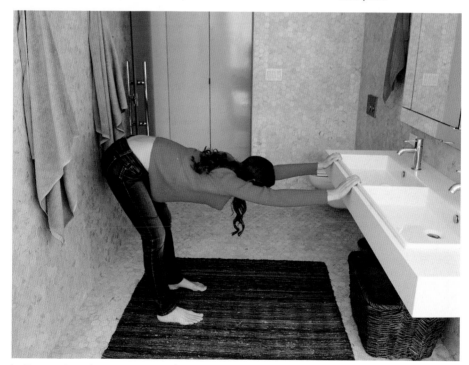

bathroom break: counter stretch

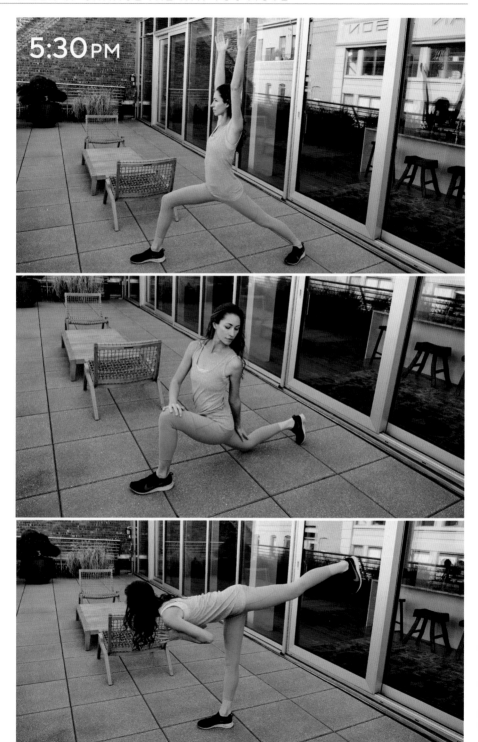

5:30PM

seasonal movement: spring rebirth yoga routine

exercises while cooking

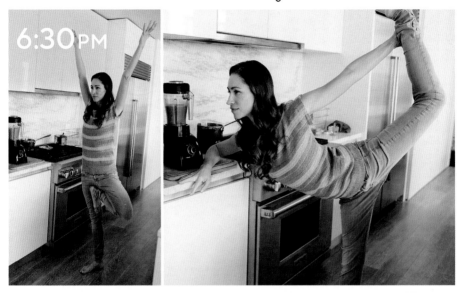

6:30PM

blender balancing act: tree pose and dancer pose

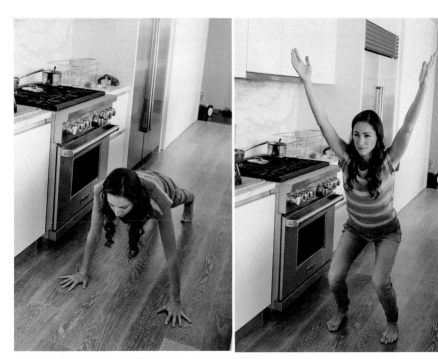

plank and chair pose wait and bake

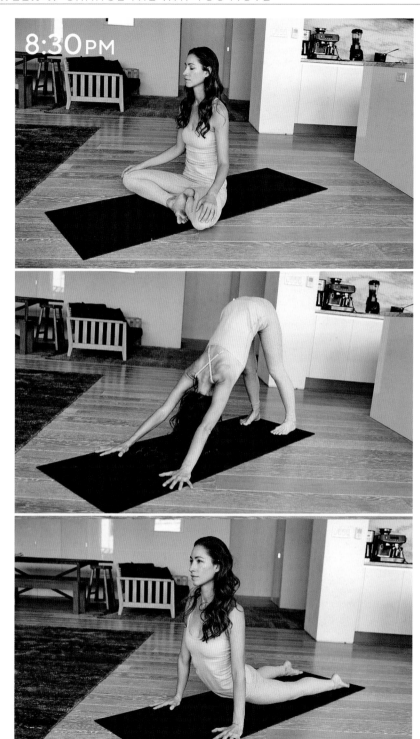

evening yoga wind-down

journal it out:
spiritual goal setting

So what are your spiritual goals? Here are some questions to ask yourself as you begin this process of reconnecting with your spiritual side. Grab your journal and jot down your answers.

- How do you want to feel when you first wake up in the morning? What changes to your life are you willing to make in order to feel this way?

- How would you characterize your interactions with others on an average day? Do you feel disconnected from people and easily irritated, or do these interactions energize you? What changes could you make to improve these interactions?

- Do you feel like you have enough time to get everything done on a typical day, or do you feel rushed and anxious? What changes could you make to feel better about what you are able to get done in a day?

- Do you feel a sense of purpose in your daily routine? If not, what changes could you make to reconnect with a sense of purpose?

- Do you feel creatively energized and "in flow" on a daily basis? If not, what changes could you make to your routine to be in flow more of the time?

Now take a look at your answers to these questions. Your responses are your spiritual goals, and the practices in this chapter—and throughout the rest of this book—are intended to get you closer to achieving these goals.

Meditation

The benefits of meditation are well documented. We all know by now that a daily meditation practice can reduce our stress, boost our creativity and productivity, benefit our physical health, and improve our mood. And yet, with all these benefits, how many of us really commit to a daily meditation practice and stick with it? If meditation were an energy drink or a supplement, we would all be buying it and gulping it down, no matter the cost. We are so caught up in our fast-paced and fast-cure lifestyles that we don't think we have even 10 minutes in a day to simply sit with ourselves. One of the many benefits of meditation is that the more regularly you practice, the easier it is to keep that practice going. You get hooked on the good feeling that the practice brings, and you keep coming back for more. The challenge is getting started and keeping it up long enough to get hooked. It may help you to know that having a specific reason for meditating—like wanting to be slower to anger in arguments with your partner—is useful for sustaining the practice. Having a specific reason to meditate gives you stronger motivation to keep it up than simply knowing you *should* be meditating.

When establishing a meditation practice, don't get caught up in externals. Don't worry about whether you are meditating at the right time of day or wearing the right clothes. All that matters is that you have a place to sit quietly, comfortably, and without interruption for at least 10 minutes a day. Is it better to meditate for longer than 10 minutes a day? Perhaps; there's some disagreement among different systems of meditation on exactly how long you should do it to reap the most benefits. But the bottom line is that having a regular meditation practice is more important than the exact amount of time you spend meditating each day. My preference is to meditate first thing in the morning, before everyone in our house wakes up, to avoid being interrupted, and I'll also sneak in an afternoon session when I can find a moment alone, even if it means locking myself in the bathroom!

Something very cool to keep in mind when starting a meditation practice is that meditating is something great you can do for your body that doesn't involve dieting or leaving the house to go to the gym. Meditation activates the vagus nerve, which quiets stress and may defeat disease. Vagus nerve action has been linked to benefits in people with migraine headaches, inflammatory bowel disease, depression, arthritis, and many other common ailments. The vagus nerve is tied to the stress hormone cortisol, the digestive hormone ghrelin, the amount of inflammation the immune system produces, and many other internal processes that shape our well-being.

Popular stress-inducing workouts, the ones that involve screaming and scrunching your face, are almost impossible to perform without setting off a stress response (the opposite of vagus nerve activation and the relaxation response). When your body is in a stress state, it also affects the way your body consumes energy—it is impossible to digest properly and healthy eating choices become much more difficult to make. So you may want to consider skipping that punishing workout, because it perpetuates a destructive cycle that keeps you calorie counting and farther away from your goal of well-being.

Meditation is a workout for your brain that activates an area of the cerebral cortex called the insula, which plays a role in diverse functions related to emotion and self-regulation, including pain, love, cravings, and addiction. Meditation has gained popularity among recovering addicts who have found that it's an effective way of controlling their addictive impulses. The insula also facilitates our concept of self-awareness in the brain. The more you stimulate your insula through meditation, the more you strengthen this area of your brain. When we meditate, the area of the insula literally lights up and is "activated," similarly to how we would think of activating our core with the plank position in a workout. Research on the functioning of the insula and the vagus nerve is nowhere near complete, but the findings thus far on the neurological benefits of meditation are too strong to ignore.

One last little analogy before we dive in. Your current morning routine might include taking a shower, brushing your teeth, getting dressed, and having some breakfast before heading out the door. Meditation should also become one of these essential parts of your morning routine. It shouldn't be something that you squeeze in only when you have some extra time in the morning. If you started your day without showering or brushing your teeth, you would probably feel a bit off, right? The same should be true for your morning meditation practice, once you have made it a habit. Morning meditation has become just as important to me as a daily shower. You could, of course, get through the day without a shower, but you wouldn't feel right. The same goes for meditation—without it, you'll survive, but you won't thrive.

MORNING MEDITATION: GETTING IN A GROOVE AND MAKING IT LAST

Morning is a great time to practice meditation because it can set up how your whole day will go. It might not have the power to change what will happen in your day ("might" being the key word here). But it will change how you react to the circumstances that show up for you, and it will help you to adjust your reactions in the best possible way. So let's get your morning set up right, and then we can chat a bit about repeating the same magic at another point in the day, maybe mid- or late afternoon, or right before bed.

You can meditate just about anywhere. I went through a phase where I liked to meditate in bed, as soon as I woke up. I would literally sit up after my alarm went off and meditate for 10 minutes right there before starting my day. A challenge to meditating from bed, however, is that you may find yourself starting to think about all the things you need to do to start your day, rather than meditating with your mind clear. It is still beneficial to sit and breathe while thinking about these things, but if heading into the shower and getting dressed first feels more natural for you, go for that, then meditate.

Another option is to keep a yoga mat on the floor by your bed. This is where I do my meditation lately, post-shower. Also, just a note that it's okay to allow yourself to change up where you meditate in the morning. If you feel like you must have an altar, or special objects to get you in the mood for meditation, those things are all fine, but completely unnecessary. For me, simplicity is key—the answers and magic are inside.

Now, here's the thing: The *how* of meditation is the simple part. All you have to do is sit. But the stuff that comes up while you are sitting there is the challenge. There will be moments when you simply can't quiet your mind, when you want to stop what you're doing, grab your phone, eat breakfast, or start your day. There will be moments of frustration when you decide you must not be meditating "right," that it's not working. There will also be moments when things feel okay or even awesome. Whatever experience you may have during a given meditation session, I can assure you that you aren't alone in having experienced it. A meditation session isn't "good" or "bad." Whether the things that come up for you while meditating are incredibly frustrating or completely blissful, every time you sit down to meditate, there is benefit to your body and mind.

STAY MOVEABLE

A mistake we commonly make while meditating is trying to sit perfectly still and statue-like. Rather than trying to sit in an awkward-feeling posture or pose because it's what you have decided that meditation should look like, sit comfortably. This is most important. Sitting comfortably doesn't mean you have to be cross-legged with your knees resting close to the floor. For many of us, a cross-legged seat on the floor is incredibly uncomfortable. For others, it's the most natural thing in the world. If sitting on the couch is most comfortable, do that. If sitting with your back against a wall is most comfortable, do that. If sitting on your heels in a kneeling position is better for your hips, do that.

You are a unique individual with a body that is important to respect and work with. Fighting yourself physically is never a good idea. You'll only lose. When we take meditation too seriously, we end up contorting ourselves into a position or posture that doesn't serve us. The reality is that meditation is a process. You are the magic. When you are comfortable, you can access the good stuff.

MANTRA OR NO MANTRA?

A mantra—from the Sanskrit *man*, meaning "mind," and *tra*, meaning "transport"—is a word or phrase repeated during meditation that's believed to have healing power and is used to help the meditator access spiritual states of consciousness. A mantra also gives the mind something to do during meditation, a way to focus. Hindu and Buddhist traditions use a mantra like the popular "om" to clear the mind. Transcendental meditation gives each practitioner their own individual mantra to focus on. You can choose a mantra on your own and essentially teach yourself. You can also meditate mantra-free, focusing on your breath instead, which is what I do in my personal practice.

3 simple
meditation practices

Here are three simple starter meditation practices to have in your toolbox. I like to think of incorporating healing practices into your life as being a bit like learning a new language. Before you can read and write in your new language, you must master the building blocks of vocabulary and grammar. These simple starter practices are your building blocks. Once you have mastered them, you will be able to move on to writing on your own, and before you know it, you will have become a poet.

BREATH-BODY CONNECTION

Breath-body connection is my favorite meditation practice, and it's the one I use most. I love how simple and effective it is. This practice is all about going along for the ride of your breath. This practice involves getting comfortable, allowing yourself to be moveable, and paying attention to your breath as it lifts and carries your body upward as you inhale, and then relaxes and lowers your body as you exhale. In the course of our busy lives, we often forget the importance of softening and tapping into the power of our breath. When we are rigid and tense, there is no room for our breath to do its magic.

As you engage in this practice, picture yourself as a flower expanding with the light of the sun in the morning, and then softening and turning inward as the light fades at night. Or picture yourself as a wave gathering energy and momentum as you inhale, and then rolling into shore as you exhale.

1. Sit comfortably. Close your eyes. Take a moment to settle in, shift position, and release any lingering tightness in your body. Breathe deeply as you gently start to sway from side to side, letting your head and neck go along for the ride.

2. Let your body soften. Inhale deeply, expanding upward and outward like a rainbow, and allowing yourself to hover for a moment at the top of your inhale. Then exhale deeply, relaxing downward and outward, until you have entirely released your breath. Stay with this for a while.

3. Continue to inhale and exhale deeply, growing and then softening, for 10 breaths. Try to clear your mind and focus only on your breath. Your thoughts will inevitably wander, and when they do, guide your attention back to your breath.

4. When you are ready to end this practice, allow your body to begin to sway again, from side to side, in any direction that feels good to you. Continue with this until your body is ready to return to stillness. Now open your eyes and take care as you go about the rest of your day.

WHO AM I?

I learned this simple and profound meditation from my friend Mallika Chopra, Deepak's daughter, who learned it from him when she was a kid. It involves asking yourself three simple questions while meditating: "Who am I? What do I want? How can I serve?" Mallika's story of learning this meditation with her dad as a kid is so funny. As she describes it, Deepak would ask Mallika and her brother, Gotham, these three questions, and they would respond with answers like tickets to a basketball game, or a new bike, and only as time went on did they get to the deeper stuff! Happiness. Health. Love.

I like to practice this meditation either on its own, or after a bit of movement in the morning, as a kind of cool-down as I set my intention for the day. It can be very powerful to repeat this every day for Week 1 and to keep track of how your answers to these questions change.

1. Start in a comfortable position. Close your eyes. Settle here and soften. Start to deepen your breath, inhaling and exhaling, and let your breath start to move you. Move in any way that feels good for you.

2. When you are ready, let yourself sway toward a calm and neutral place. Settle here for a moment. Keep those deep breaths rolling through you. If you notice your attention wandering, guide it back to your breath.

3. In your mind, ask yourself, "Who am I?" Don't try too hard to find an answer. Simply ask and see what comes up for you.

4. In your mind, ask yourself, "What do I want?" Again, no need to struggle for an answer. Simply notice what comes up.

5. In your mind, ask yourself, "How can I serve?" Let the question roll through you and notice how you feel. Let yourself settle here for a bit.

6. Feel free to repeat this series of questions once or twice more. When you are ready, allow yourself to settle, and open your eyes.

WRITE IT OUT AND COME BACK

It's common to find yourself distracted by various thoughts or ideas during meditation. I often find myself in a situation where a really cool, creative idea pops up and I just can't stand the thought of losing it, so I hold on to it for the rest of my meditation and miss out on all the good stuff that might have happened if I was not distracted. Some meditation techniques say that you should just keep trying to return to your breath when these thoughts creep up, but I prefer a different remedy. I've started keeping a notebook nearby while I meditate, to record these just-won't-quit thoughts and ideas.

The meditation part of this practice is similar to the practices outlined on page 81—but when a thought drifts in that just won't quit, you stop to write it down, and then come back to your meditation practice. I hope this little trick gives you the freedom to feel more connected and relaxed during your meditation time.

MEDITATION LATER IN THE DAY

Once you've mastered a 10- to 20-minute morning meditation session, your next step is to add a second, shorter 5- to 10-minute meditation practice later in the day. It's a great way to keep the good vibes going. I find that the best time for a second meditation session is after lunch, at around two or three P.M. Whatever you can fit in is beneficial. If you can't find time in the afternoon and right before bed is the only time you have for yourself, then that works, too. The best time to meditate is a time that is convenient for you, because—let's be honest—if it's not convenient, you're not going to do it. If you have trouble sleeping, meditating just before bed can be a great habit to get into, helping you to wind down and release the day's tension.

Slowing Down

Our culture would lead us to believe that slowing down is only acceptable later in life. We've all been at family gatherings where we've heard older relatives say things like, "Well, I'm slowing down these days, but hanging in there." And this is allowed, once we hit a certain age. Otherwise, we're supposed to stay crazy busy, working hard, barely resting, right? Deciding to slow down and simply do less during the years when we're expected to be our busiest and most productive is frowned upon. We fear scrutiny, lack of respect, or that we won't be able to pick up where we left off when we are ready to gear up again. We experience massive fear of missing out. Prioritizing our well-being over achieving is seen as lazy by modern standards. Interestingly, the act of radical self-care might just be the magic ingredient that leads us to more profound work and creativity.

Many of us pack our schedules during the week, thinking we can save slowing down and recharging for the weekends, or for vacation. Of course, it doesn't work this way. Because after we've been on the treadmill all week, we collapse in a heap when the weekend arrives. Spending your weekend on the couch in sweats, eating junk, and binge-watching Netflix is not a healthy recharge. This sort of yo-yo lifestyle is a guaranteed recipe for burnout, and for our bodies rebelling against us and getting sick.

Instead of the kind of vicious cycle I've just described, we need to find balance. We must do that by slowing down, and we need to stop stigmatizing slowness. Here are some very simple, manageable ways to do that.

PRACTICES FOR SLOWING DOWN

A sustainable pace of life doesn't have to mean living off the grid, although that might be a lot of fun for a while if you are the adventurous type. Here are a few simple practices to add into your routine that will help you with slowing down and reconnecting with what you truly value.

Nature walks—I've already discussed the many benefits of outdoor walking in this book, but really, I can't emphasize this one enough. I make sure to walk outside every day, no matter the time of year or the weather. I love watching the birds, getting close to the grass and trees, and getting on intimate terms with nature. If nature is your backyard, that is wonderful, but if you live in the city or in a suburban area, getting outside is just as useful. If you live in a more populated area, seeing other people on your walks can also be great for your well-being, especially when you allow yourself to acknowledge them.

DIY bathroom spa—This is another restorative practice with incredible benefits, which we often forget about. A good hot soak with some Epsom salts, bubble bath, or your favorite essential oils can be incredibly calming and rejuvenating. I like to take a long bath before bed two or three times a week, and I swear by this practice for winding down. If you don't have a tub (yes, I've lived in those apartments, too), you can gain similar benefits by taking some extra time for yourself in the bathroom with a good foot soak involving your essential oils and Epsom salts. I like to spend some time sitting on my bathroom floor doing simple self-shiatsu exercises like leaning my elbow into my upper inner thigh, a great practice for balancing yin, or softer energy. If you feel like you are constantly doing and performing in the world, you are expressing your yang energy frequently. It's important to work toward balance of our doing/yang and receiving/yin energy for overall well-being. This was a practice I did regularly when trying to conceive Daisy. It's not exclusively related to reproductive health, but it is wonderful for allowing your whole nervous system to slow down.

Quiet time—I love enforcing quiet time, whether I'm alone or with someone else, as long as they are up for it. This is a practice I came up with out of a need to bring a sense of calm to my busiest days. Today I practice at least 10 minutes of designated quiet time at some point every day. Sometimes I'll announce "quiet time" when I'm in the car with Mike on our way to the grocery store, or when we're on our way to pick up Daisy from school. He thinks it's hilarious that I do this, but he also appreciates the sense of calm he gains from these designated periods of quiet. Usually, after we've taken a break for quiet, we have more meaningful things to say to one another.

how to practice shiatsu on your own

Shiatsu is normally done with a partner, but you can also practice alone. We naturally touch ourselves to soothe aches and pains, and this tendency is the basis of self-shiatsu. Here are few shiatsu pressure points you can try stimulating on your own.

- Dig an elbow into your inner thigh while sitting cross-legged on the floor to promote relaxation.
- Apply pressure to the outside of your thigh to promote release of control.
- Press with your thumb into the middle of the sole of your foot to promote a reset of balance between tiredness and overexcitedness.

You can also practice self-shiatsu by paying attention to which areas of your body are holding tightness and tension, and focusing there. Bring some pressure with a thumb, elbow, or hand to these areas. Take a few deep breaths and notice any changes. The more you learn about the meridians, the more you can play around, but the basics are always the same: relax, breathe, lean.

Pleasure reading—Another obvious one, but it's something we don't set aside enough time for. Reading is fun, informative, and an opportunity to escape into a whole new world for a while.

Books are magic, and if you are out of the habit of reading regularly, it is great to reestablish this practice. I'm not talking about skimming the news on your phone. I mean reading an actual book. I also think it's important to push yourself to read beyond the categories that you naturally gravitate toward based on your interests. If you are reading this book, chances are you tend to gravitate toward wellness and health books. That's great, but it might also be fun and expansive to pick up a classic like *Frankenstein*, or an inspiring memoir or biography about someone from a different time. Great books are like great people. One will lead you to the next, and you'll form your own beautiful story of exploring along the way.

Living with Intention

It is impossible to live mindfully and to interact with the world in a way that is mindful if you aren't at peace with yourself. The self-care practices we have been discussing in this book are like prep work, essential for grounding yourself so that when stressful situations arise, you can respond in a way that's calm and productive, rather than being tossed around in the moment. The goal is to be able to stay balanced and calm in moments of stress, just as you would in moments of ease. Living mindfully isn't about passively accepting injustice when stressful moments arise. It's about being better prepared internally, so you can respond with clarity and keep your well-being intact. Think of all your self-care, meditation, goal setting, and journaling as preparation for these real-life moments.

setting an intention for your day

This is a great practice to embrace for focusing your mind and preparing before you start your day. By setting an intention for the day, you begin with a vision of how you want your day to go, so when obstacles arise or challenging decisions need to be made, you have a positive mental state guiding your actions. Of course, you will drift away from your intention throughout the day—that is inevitable—but the power of intention remains present in our being once we've set it.

A great time to set your intention for the day is either before or after your morning meditation. And if your meditation is just not happening one morning, no need to beat yourself up—you can still set your intention as you get ready for your day, maybe while you're in the shower or as you get dressed.

1. Take a few deep breaths and imagine how you want to feel throughout your day. Bring to mind the actions you would like to participate in throughout your day.

2. Set your intention for your day. It should just be a simple sentence about how you ideally want to show up and react to the things you encounter that day. These are some of my favorite evergreen intentions to get you going:

   - I intend to connect from my heart in all I do.

   - I intend to appreciate what I have.

- I intend to listen to my body and respond to its needs.

- I intend to slow down enough so I can hear my intuition.

- I intend to listen to understand others the best I can.

These simple statements become like a relationship carrying you through your day. Your intention will deepen over the course of your day, as you use it as a guiding light for the experiences and decisions you face. Setting an intention for your day makes you a magnet for great things that will come your way and gives you the mental space to interact with the world on your own terms. Doing good for yourself and for others becomes easy, fun, and joyful instead of a chore. And dealing with stressful situations with a sense of calm and confidence becomes second nature.

When setting an intention for your day, it is also important to think about the emotions that you want to feel over the course of that day. This will help you to navigate days that you know will be particularly challenging and that you will need to confront with an extra dose of gratitude or grace. Let an emotion that you want to feel float into your mind during your morning meditation, and hold that word in your mind. Try not to pick an emotion before it comes to you. Just let it float into your consciousness. Some examples of emotions that might bubble up for you include:

Joy

Harmony

Compassion

Healing

Ease

Okay, now that you've got a handle on what daily intention setting entails, here are a few of my favorite, go-to, feeling-based intention-setting practices. These don't have to happen in the morning. They can be used all day long to keep you centered, focused, and calm!

MINDFUL MOMENT PRACTICE

Even when we manage to squeeze in morning meditation and a healthy breakfast, we may still find ourselves losing our cool during moments of stress. But we can preempt these inevitable, stressful moments by taking short breathing breaks, which I call "Mindful Moments," throughout the course of the day. The best time for a "Mindful Moment" is when you have at least 10 free minutes between activities: waiting for a meeting to begin, standing in line, commuting on the train, or enjoying some quiet time at home alone before your family returns. Instead of grabbing your phone and scrolling during these free moments, take the opportunity to return to yourself.

- *Get comfortable.* If you are standing, widen your stance a bit and soften your knees and joints so you are moveable. If you are sitting in a chair, adjust so that your feet are resting on the floor and you are relaxed. Close your eyes and notice what's going on inside. Listen to your breath.

- *Return to your intention.* If you set an intention for your day during your morning meditation, return to it now. If you haven't yet set an intention for your day, set one now—but don't force it. Embrace a thought or feeling that comes to you naturally in this moment, and that reflects who you want to be throughout this particular day. Stay easy with yourself. Repeat your intention silently to yourself as you breathe deeply, in and out.

- *Let your intention go.* After 10 minutes or so, let your intention go. Know that it will stay with you throughout your day, as you face moments of stress and challenge. Take a few more deep breaths before gently opening your eyes and easing back into your day.

People Who Are Living It Right

I'd like to introduce you to some friends whom I consider my role models for how to live spiritually, mindfully, and gracefully in the world. We all have people like this in our lives, who serve as our shining examples for how to live. These people for you could be the barista who makes your coffee, the security guard who greets you at work in the morning, or someone in the public eye whom you admire. These spiritual guides are all around us, and we can learn from them if we slow down and pay attention. Similar to the way that meditation open us up to greater creativity and intuition, when we embrace the everyday wisdom of people we admire, we live spiritually richer lives.

MALLIKA CHOPRA
Author and Entrepreneur, on Why You Need a Reason to Meditate

Mallika Chopra is a good friend of mine, someone I turn to for support, advice, and fun! Daughter of Deepak, she is the founder of Intent.com, a platform that connects people from around the world through social media in order to improve their lives, their communities, and the planet. Whenever I have the opportunity to hang out with Mallika, I take it. I just love to soak up her wisdom.

What is the secret to sticking with a meditation practice?

For many, establishing a meditation practice can truly be difficult. We live in a hyperstimulated world where distractions and busyness follow us, despite our best intentions. The key to meditating regularly is knowing *why you want to do it*. Intellectually, we understand the benefits. There is tremendous research on the physical, emotional, and overall health benefits to the practice. Meditation can help you sleep better, feel less stress, improve your health, and connect more deeply with others. But knowing why you want to meditate will help you stick with it.

What is the main motivating factor for your meditation practice? How can we find motivation when we fall out of the habit?

Since I have been meditating since I was nine years old, I can look back over many decades now and see how the practice has affected me. There have been years where I meditated twice a day, morning, and afternoon, and then years when I didn't meditate at all! Today I meditate once a day for 15 minutes. I can see how the times when I thought I was too busy to meditate, I was generally more scattered, stressed, and overwhelmed by life. When I meditated more regularly, I was calmer, more focused and successful, and happier. Meditation has proved to be the anchor that keeps me grounded, healthier, and able to have more perspective.

For me, it is often difficult to get back in the habit of doing something—whether it is meditation, yoga, exercising, or eating differently. My approach is to start with baby steps, and do what I can do, but make it daily. So that may begin with 5 minutes every day of meditating instead of 15 minutes, or one sun salutation instead of my whole yoga routine. Once I return to my practice, I see how much I yearn for it when I miss it.

Are there particular times during the day, or special places, that you recommend for meditating?

Meditate in your favorite chair at home, or in a park or church near your office. Find a place where you feel safe, and where you won't be distracted. Try to set aside the same time every day to practice. For example, I used to meditate every day before picking up my girls from school. It became part of my afternoon routine, after I had my cup of tea. And when my girls got older and the schedule changed, I adjusted my meditation time to midmorning after I had done some work. Be flexible, but also set the intention to do it daily.

Is intention setting something we should be doing daily along with meditation?

You don't need to meditate to set an intention. But setting a daily intent after your meditation practice can be fun and powerful. I like to think of daily intents as "micro-intents," anchors for the day that help you focus more on what is specifically important to you at a particular time. Micro-intents can be things like connecting with a friend or spending time soaking in the sun. They don't have to be life-changing. They should be fun and about feeling better in the here and now.

How can "micro-intents" help us to further our larger goals?

Micro-intents can help you to define and pursue larger life goals that at times may seem overwhelming. Larger life intentions often involve thinking about who you aspire to be, how you want to live, and how you can serve. These take time—incubation—to be realized and incorporated into your life. It is in your meditation practice that you will begin to know more deeply your larger life intentions and destiny. If you have a daily meditation practice, it is nice to incorporate a micro-intent at the end to just recognize what you need for that particular day. Start the morning thinking about how you want to feel—maybe it's more energetic or connected or peaceful—and have fun seeing how you can make it happen throughout the day.

How can we find purpose in our lives when things feel off?

First, it is important to recognize that life is a messy journey. It is normal and natural to have ups and downs, to feel confused, to feel lonely and disconnected. Resilience involves having the emotional tools to recalibrate and respond in new ways to ever-changing internal and external situations. My primary tool has always been a regular meditation practice and intention setting. But at different times in your life, you may need to try new things, as well. Recently, I have been reconnecting with college friends after falling out of touch during the early years of parenting my kids. I've realized that these friendships are some of my most precious, and I now make a conscious effort to see these friends at least once a year. This has been one of the most powerful reenergizers for me!

RABBI JONATHAN BLAKE
on Shifting Your Mind-Set from "Serve Us" to "Service"

Rabbi Jonathan Blake first walked into our yoga studio to take a class years ago, and not long after, I jokingly asked him if he would be Strala's unofficial rabbi. He thought that was sweet, and accepted! Always thinking of others, every time he comes in for a class, he brings someone with him who needs yoga in their life. Jonathan's connection to his spirituality and his commitment to his own well-being and the well-being of others is inspiring, and contagious.

What do you do to stay mentally, physically, and spiritually balanced?

The way I look at it, compartmentalizing our mental, physical, and spiritual selves, which we all do, pretty much all the time, does us a tremendous disservice. Body, mind, spirit—it's all one. We need to nourish all of it, holistically, to grow our humanity and to become the most fully realized version of ourselves that we can be. And, truth be told, we'd do well to visualize *self* as part of a whole, too. After all, there is no such thing as a "self" that is totally self-contained or separate from its environment. The notion of the "self" is an illusion. Professor Daniel Matt, who recently produced a monumental translation of the Zohar, the great work of Jewish mysticism, puts it this way: "Just because we have words for all the parts of a tree . . . does not mean that a tree really has all those parts. All our names are, likewise, only arbitrarily superimposed on what is, in truth, one great seamless reality." Who are we to say where the branch ends and the bud begins? Where the trunk ends and the roots begin? Where the roots end and the soil begins? Who are we to say where you end and the universe begins?

When I was in seminary, I studied with the late Bonia Shur, a professor and composer of sacred Jewish music. He would lead us in a chant: *Everything is connected. Everything is connected. Everything is connected.* And this is what I believe.

Do you have a daily practice that guides you? How does this practice inform your long-term goals?

Meditation can be clarifying. That's a tool just for me, alone in a chair, that provides just enough disruption from the noise (the noise in my schedule and the noise cluttering my head) to break unhealthy thought patterns and open up new pathways for creative thinking and a calmer approach to everything else. My life partner and wife, Kelly, is a steadfast guide. She is my sounding board, counselor, teacher, and supporter. She keeps me honest. It is good to have someone like this in life, because, as a friend once told me, "It's hard being a person." Having another person makes it a little bit easier to be a person. That's why I've committed, as well, to weekly psychotherapy, and why I meet regularly with an executive leadership coach. Because not everything needs to be tackled alone. It's good to ask for help.

As for goals—goals are good but can be overrated. I don't think I've ever spent any time thinking about more than the next five years, and even that is a stretch. Ram Dass was right to remind us to "Be here now." Learning to cultivate flexibility and responsiveness to changing circumstances is, in my experience, a better life skill than having a great five-year plan. After all, Darwin's oft-misquoted idea about "survival of the fittest" gives no absolute advantage to physical strength, or big brains, or sex appeal. It *does* give an advantage to beings who are adaptable, particularly under stress.

What's the biggest thing we can do to stay connected to our purpose?

Give of yourself to others. It's so simple, and so easy to forget. Right now, my wife is helping to steer a volunteer effort at my synagogue to resettle a family of refugee women who have fled genocide and military conflict in the Central African Republic. Two African sisters, ages twenty-six and thirty-eight, arrived in our community this past spring, each carrying to America a suitcase, a positive attitude, and a history of trauma. Within weeks of working with our volunteers—learning their first English words, attending their first community dinner, figuring out how to shop for groceries on a very tight budget and government benefits, setting up their first apartment—one described their welcome to the community as "seeing God's smile." How do you think that made Kelly feel? How do you think you'd feel?

How can we find our spiritual community and live with intention?

Start with what you have to give to others. This could be your time, your talent, your ideas, your recipes, your songs, your way of moving through the world. You want to find your spiritual community? Stop asking how you can find a place to meet your spiritual needs and instead connect where you can give joyfully to others. It's the difference in mind-set between "serve us" and "service." Find that place where you can give, and everything else will follow: joy, purpose, and transformation. What are you waiting for?

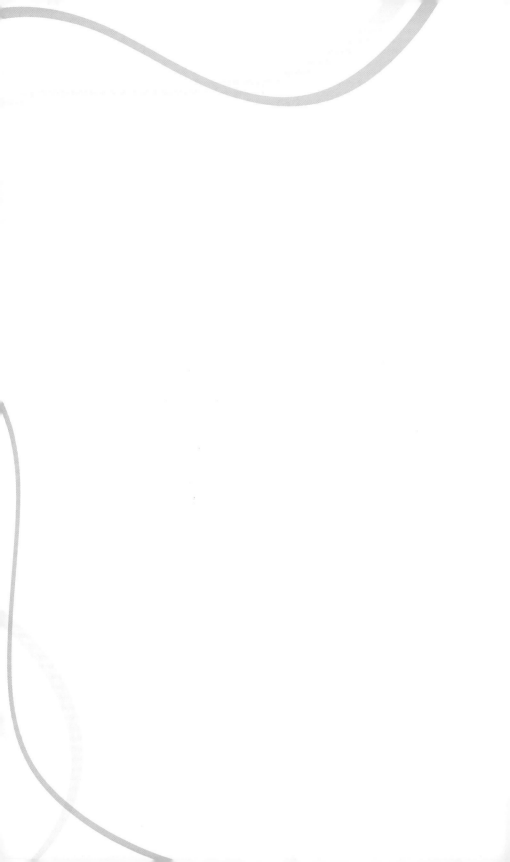

clean
body

3

hit the reset:

change the way you eat

Don't eat anything your great-grandmother wouldn't recognize as food.
—Michael Pollan

When you feel mentally and spiritually balanced, with a settled mind as your foundation, it becomes much easier to make choices that are good for your body. This is why it's essential to achieve mental clarity and spiritual calm before embarking on the Clean Body phase of your journey. When your mind is stressed, your entire body is stressed. It doesn't matter how much green juice you consume, or how many yoga classes you take. Stress builds up in the body, taxing the immune system, preparing your body for battle, and ultimately making you feel sick, sluggish, and out of balance. Health is multifactorial, a cocktail of our genetics, our lifestyle choices, and environmental stresses and toxins. But there is a lot that we can control when it comes to our health, by making good diet and lifestyle choices, and controlling certain elements of our environment.

As we turn to caring for the physical body with nourishing and detoxifying foods and exercise, let's be sure not to lose sight of what we learned about maintaining mental and spiritual balance during Weeks 1 and 2. It is essential to keep mind and body in harmony throughout this journey. It's also important to remember that your body's needs are constantly changing, depending on the events of your life, your life stage, and the seasons. You can support your life stage for optimal well-being by making informed food choices instead of being a victim to your existing food habits. Eating in harmony with nature and the seasons helps support your body's natural rhythm and balance. There is no one size or one meal that fits all, but the more you understand the process and the nourishing power of food, the more you can choose and enjoy the most appropriate meals to nourish your needs.

We are going to shift the way you think about food and nourishing your body through the practices in this chapter. You are going to change the way you eat—and that is always a challenge. It's rare to hear someone say, "I'm on this new diet and I feel so satisfied and happy." We more typically associate dieting with feeling hungry, deprived, and moody, with battling our cravings, and with struggling to break old habits and forge new ones. The detoxes, recipes, and practices in this chapter are designed to overhaul your current bad habits and to forge lasting new ones that will better support your goals. They aren't designed to restrict or deprive you, but you will most likely feel challenged in some way. Whether that's physical, mental, spiritual, or emotional completely depends on your specific health situation and your starting point. As you progress through this chapter, try to keep your larger goals in mind when you are feeling challenged. At moments of frustration, know that you are headed somewhere great. At moments when you are feeling energized, recognize that this feeling can be sustainable, rather than fleeting. In order to stick with this phase, stay connected to how you want the food you eat to make you feel—more energetic, less foggy, with improved strength and mood.

Whenever you feel stress and tension arise, return to your breath and to the mental and spiritual practices in chapters 1 and 2 of this book. We're aiming for lasting transformation, change that comes from the inside, not a quick fix that will allow you to drop a few pounds or fit into your skinny jeans. This is about wholeness and restoring the real you.

Nourishing Habits

Ideally, we want to think about food in terms of true nourishment and wellness, as opposed to fixed goals like calorie counts or numbers on the scale—but that can be difficult. Even when we try to shift our thinking, old patterns of thought regarding things like ideal weight and size creep in uninvited. It will take some dedication and discipline to point your actions toward true well-being and away from body comparison, but the energy you'll gain from steering yourself in the right direction will be worth it. Direct your attention toward building nourishing habits that will support your health, and away from fixed numbers, sizes, and comparisons.

It's important to start where you are and be honest with yourself about the way you are currently feeding your body, and how this is serving you mentally, physically, and spiritually. It's easy to lose touch with our eating habits. They are such an intrinsic part of who we are that we are not always aware of them. But once we are ready to make a real change, we must slow down and take a closer look. Unhealthy eating habits, like all destructive habits, can be incredibly hard to break. In this section, we're going to work toward replacing our old, harmful habits with habits that actually serve us and make us feel great.

journal it out

As we begin, consider this set of questions regarding your eating habits and jot down the answers that come to mind. Those answers will inform your goals for this stage of your journey.

- How do you typically feel when you wake up in the morning? How does your diet contribute to this feeling?

- On a typical day, do you rush through most of your meals, so that you can quickly get back to your work or activities?

- Do you experience anxiety surrounding food? Does thinking about what you will eat make you worried or stressed?

- Are grocery shopping and cooking a joy or are they dreaded tasks? Do you enjoy preparing your own food, or is your life too hectic to cook?

- Do you eat meals with others, engaged in conversation and the act of eating? Do you prefer to eat alone? Do you eat in front of the computer or while scrolling through your phone?

- Are you addicted to stimulating foods like sugar and caffeine to keep you going throughout the day, or to foods with a particular taste or texture (salty, crunchy, etc.)?

- What time of day do your cravings kick in? Do you experience a midday slump and crave sugar and caffeine? Do you crave foods late at night that you wouldn't eat during the day?

- Do you tend to overindulge in junk when you aren't feeling so great, mentally or physically?

- And the big question: If you could wave a magic wand and wake up tomorrow morning having the perfect relationship with food, what would that look like?

And as you contemplate this "big question," let me also offer a bit of help to get you started. Here is how I would like to feel throughout a day of true nourishment:

- I would like to wake up early in the morning, with lots of energy, not overly sleepy, and feeling ready for the day.

- I would like to feel energized all morning long, have time for myself to meditate and practice before the rest of the day begins.

- I would like to feel hungry and excited for a colorful lunch around midday and not feel sluggish after eating.

- I would like to have energy and inspiration to carry me through the afternoon.

- I would like to feel calm at night and find it easy to wind down for a restful sleep.

Okay, now take the time to write out how you would like food to make you feel on a typical day. This should ideally give you a clear path of where you are right now, and where you'd like to point yourself throughout this section. Let your imagination run wild: write out how you would really like to feel, even if a part of you thinks it is very far away from the reality of your situation.

Now that you've got your list, it's time to get started! Here are the three phases of your Diet Detox:

Embrace East Meets West: We'll focus on soaking up the principles of Ayurveda and modifying this ancient practice to promote healthy eating in modern life.

Eat Clean and Eat Well: We'll establish Clean Body Food Rules that will do your body right.

Be in Your Body: We'll focus on loving and nourishing your body, enjoying being in your body, and establishing a healthy body image.

As with the previous chapters, the goal is to dive into each week fully, so that each of these practices become a part of you as we add on. And following this seven-day reset, you will continue to incorporate these practices into your daily routine.

EMBRACE EAST MEETS WEST

We're living in the age of the "wellness product" and the "wellness retreat," but there's a pretty big disconnect between what we know, intellectually, to be true about wellness and our actual behavior. Much of this has to do with confusing external messaging we get from sources like the diet industry. Most of us know that eating well involves consuming whole, fresh, unprocessed foods, but the diet industry throws us off course, making things more complicated than they need to be and misleading us into thinking that we need to eliminate entire food groups or take other extreme measures to be fit and healthy. We know, deep down, that fad dieting is not the path to health. But it can be tough to resist the false promises and messages of the diet industry. We must learn to find our true north when it comes to the way we are eating and to tune in to our body's needs.

Instead of falling prey to diet trends, let's turn to a time-honored system of nourishing the body: Ayurveda.

A BRIEF HISTORY OF AYURVEDA

Ayurveda is a system of natural medicine that originated in India more than three thousand years ago. It is based on the idea that a delicate balance exists between the body, the mind, and the spirit, and that disease occurs when these elements are out of balance. *Ayurveda* is composed of two Sanskrit words: *ayur*, meaning "life," and *veda*, meaning "knowledge." The Ayurvedic tradition was passed down orally until around 1000 BCE, when it was inscribed as part of the Vedas, an ancient body of sacred texts. Ayurveda is known as one of the oldest developed medical systems.

Ayurveda is similar to traditional Chinese medicine (TCM), and practices like shiatsu and acupuncture, in the sense that it promotes well-being through diet and lifestyle changes that encourage energy flow, called prana in Ayurveda and chi in TCM, throughout the body. Ayurveda and TCM have long been referred to as "alternative medicine" in Western culture and relegated to the sidelines of healthcare. But we are coming to recognize the value of these systems, and today Western physicians increasingly recommend some of the principles of Ayurveda or TCM to promote health and ward off disease.

THE AYURVEDIC DIET

Although Ayurveda is an ancient practice, it is incredibly adaptable to our busy, modern lives. But consuming an Ayurvedic diet on its own is not enough—we also need to live the full process. Ayurveda is as much about coming to understand yourself—how your natural tendencies and moods interact with the seasons, the rhythms of a day, and certain foods—as it is about the foods you eat.

Ayurveda places a lot of focus on your digestive fire, or *agni* in Sanskrit. In Ayurveda, agni is essential to overall well-being. When your agni is in balance, you are able to digest food properly while ridding the body of toxins, thereby producing a clear mind. Practices that promote a strong agni include meditation, walking, eating small meals, eating your largest meal at lunchtime, and drinking ginger tea.

THE AYURVEDIC DOSHAS

In Ayurveda, there are three *doshas*, or mind-body types: *vata* (air), *pitta* (fire), and *kapha* (earth). Your physical body type tends to indicate your predominant dosha, but personality and temperament are also factors, and many of us are a combination of two doshas (bidoshic), or all three (tridoshic).

- *Vata:* Slim, willowy build. Associated with the elements of space, air, and lightness. Corresponds to a personality that is moody, impulsive, and quick to act. When vata is out of balance, sleep and digestion are disrupted. Vata is encouraged to eat on a schedule, eat earlier in the day, eat cooked foods, and manage stress and overstimulation.

- *Pitta:* Athletic or medium build. Associated with the elements of fire and water. Corresponds to a fiery, strong personality. Pitta is often intolerant of heat, has a high metabolism and a sharp analytical mind, and is very goal focused. Anything that creates too much fire sends pitta out of balance. Competitiveness can lead to anger and frustration. "Cooling" the fire through food and lifestyle helps to balance pitta. Suggestions include choosing cooling foods like salads and cucumbers.

- *Kapha:* Larger or rounder build. Associated with earth and water. Kapha tends to be slow, steady, earthy, and not easily angered. When kapha is out of balance, headaches and problems with mucus arise. Kapha also tends to get stuck in a routine and can put on weight. Kapha benefits from regular physical activity to get the heart rate up and is encouraged to limit sugar, eat more fruits and vegetables, and avoid overindulging.

But if you look at a person's size and weight alone, you miss the bigger picture. It's important to understand that one's dosha is not a fixed state—it's more of a guideline for tailoring our habits and behaviors. Our bodies are fluid, always changing based on what is happening in our lives and the seasons. Your physical health and well-being depend on your doshic balance. There are three states:

- *Balanced:* All three doshas are in harmony.

- *Increased:* One dosha is in a larger portion or aggravated state.

- *Decreased:* One dosha is in a lower-than-normal proportion or depleted state.

Whether you identify strongly with one dosha or not, you are aiming for harmony between them all, and the way to achieve this harmony is by adjusting your diet to correct imbalance, improving your lifestyle to reduce stress, and removing waste and toxins from your body with the support of Ayurvedic herbs like triphala, an herbal concoction taken as a tea to balance the doshas and detox. (Triphala has a mild laxative effect and is not safe for everyone, including pregnant women, so be sure you consult your doctor before trying triphala or any herbal remedy.)

dosha reflection

Here are some questions to ask yourself in order to discover your dosha leaning during this phase of your life. Self-diagnosing your dosha is never a perfect process, and if you have the opportunity I'd recommend seeing an Ayurvedic doctor or practitioner for more information. But these questions are a place to start, and your answers will give insight into how you can start adjusting your diet and lifestyle to bring yourself into balance. If you answer yes to more questions associated with one of the doshas than the others, you may have found your main leaning. An equal number of yeses for two could mean you are bidoshic, and an equal number of yeses for all three could mean you are tridoshic.

Vata Questions

- Do you reach for caffeine to keep you going throughout the day, rush from one thing to the next, and often start multiple projects at once?

- Are you most creative at night? Do you tend to stay up late and feel exhausted in the morning?

- Do you reach for cold foods and quick, sugary snacks like fruit, chips and crackers, and juices to keep you going?

- Do you feel like there are constantly creative ideas coming your way, and do you tend to have a hard time seeing all your ideas through?

Pitta Questions

- Is it common for you to feel joy one moment and anger the next? Do you find yourself in a lot of heated arguments?

- Does your body feel overheated sometimes?
- Do you generally feel like you have a lot of endurance and physical power, which gets you through your day?
- Do you have a lot of ambition and drive?

- Is it easy for you to love and nurture others? Do you sometimes lose yourself in caring for someone else?
- Do you feel steady, stable, and slow-moving?
- Do you feel heavy and sometimes stuck in where you are?
- Are your hands often moist?

No matter your primary dosha type, reducing stress, eating fewer processed foods, having a daily routine that includes eating your largest meal at midday, practicing meditation, and getting regular exercise are recommended for staying in balance. The following lists have recommendations for foods and drinks to consume or avoid/limit depending on your dosha type.

VATA

Imbalance Symptoms

When aggravated, vata can become depleted and experience constipation, dehydration, weight loss, disturbed sleep, anxiety, and being cold.

Avoid/Limit

Cold foods such as salads, iced drinks, and raw vegetables

Excess caffeine and sugar

Warm soups, stews, and hot cereals

Easily digestible ripe fruits

Nourishing foods with moderately heavy texture, including dairy, raw nuts, and nut butters

Mild spices like cumin, ginger, cardamom, salt, black pepper, and mustard

Chamomile, ginger, and lemon teas

Vata is prone to anxiety and drawn to fast-paced, sweaty workouts. To balance vata, yoga, meditation, and brisk walking are recommended. Go to bed early to get plenty of rest.

PITTA

When imbalanced, pitta can become irritable, self-critical, and aggressive. Symptoms of imbalance include diarrhea, overheating, excessive hunger, and heartburn.

Fermented foods, pickles, sour cream, and cheese

Oily, hot, and salty foods, and heavy fried foods

Coffee (for pittas who experience heartburn and skin rashes, and who often feel angry, irritated, or judgmental)

Cool or warm foods with moderately heavy textures

Vegetarian foods, including steamed and raw vegetables, sweet fruits, rice, wheat, and oats

Mild spices like turmeric, cardamom, and mint

Peppermint and chamomile teas

Exercise and Lifestyle

Pittas tend to have good stamina and love to work their muscles to the maximum capacity. They are drawn to boot camps, long runs and swims, and anything that pushes their body to the limit. It's suggested for pittas to take rest days. Pittas should avoid overworking and overstimulation.

KAPHA

Imbalance Symptoms

Mental and physical stagnation are signs of kapha imbalance. Symptoms of imbalance in kapha include sluggish bowels, water retention, weight gain, and excessive sleep.

Avoid/Limit

Excessive consumption of sweet, fatty, deep-fried, or salty foods

Added sugar and fats

Dairy products

A warm, light diet, including lightly cooked foods or raw fruits and vegetables

Spicy foods and strong spices like pepper, garlic, fennel, and ginger; preferred spices are cumin, fenugreek, sesame seed, and turmeric

Exercise and Lifestyle

Kaphas tend to be slow and steady and often avoid movement, but once kaphas get moving, they have the most stamina of all the doshas. Kaphas might be drawn to weight training, but they should balance that with cardio and workouts that work up a sweat. Try to avoid sleeping during the day. Keep things moving with brisk walks during the day for better sleep at night.

A regular meditation and gentle yoga practice, time in nature, and creating a daily routine are recommended for all dosha types.

---

coffee, alcohol, and ayurveda

Ayurveda teaches us that all plants serve a purpose, and coffee is best viewed as medicine. Consuming coffee might be good for some dosha types and not great for others. Overall, Ayurveda recommends keeping an eye on the effects that coffee has on you personally and deciding whether to continue as usual, reduce your intake, or cut coffee out altogether, depending on those effects. If you need coffee to feel energized, it's important to look at your quality of sleep and your activity levels during the day. For strong vata types, coffee might best be avoided and swapped out for ginger tea. Coffee can also lead to poor focus and difficulty sleeping for some vatas. Pittas might want to avoid coffee also, aside from the occasional after-breakfast cup to rev up, as it can result in overproduction of anger and gastric reflux for this type. Kaphas may benefit from the stimulating nature of coffee, and its diuretic effect might help dry up the heavy, wet nature of kapha.

Ayurveda textbooks say alcohol quickly reaches the heart and mind and that over time, alcohol consumption will create agitation and dullness. Traditional Ayurveda also says that alcohol should be consumed in moderation and that consumption must be considered in relation to the qualities of the food or drink taken with it, the consumer's age, their strength of digestion, their current state of health, the season of the year, and even the time of day. Vata's suggestions for alcohol are a low-alcohol sweet beer or sweet or plum wine for a calming effect. Pitta's suggestion is a bitter or astringent white wine like chardonnay for cooling. Kapha's suggestion is a dry red wine to stimulate fires. The Ayurvedic serving size for wine is 2 to 4 ounces, compared to the standard 5-ounce Western pour. Overall, Ayurveda recommends honoring your body, your history, and your circumstances when choosing whether to consume alcohol or not. Observe your reaction, and adjust your choices accordingly for optimal vitality.

TRANSLATING AYURVEDA FOR OUR MODERN LIVES

I discovered Ayurveda as a young yoga instructor in my early twenties, and I was initially quite confused about how to bring this ancient practice into my life in a way that was practical and respectful to the tradition it descended from. There I was, a young woman from the Midwest, living in New York City, wrapped in a sari, burning incense, and cooking lentils, alongside peers and teachers in the yoga world who seemed to be doing the same, some even going so far as to change their names to Sanskrit ones. I never want to judge my fellow seekers, but this felt off to me, and I knew I needed to find a better way.

Ayurveda has become a wellness trend, and today there are Western Ayurvedic experts who head off to India regularly to further their studies. This is certainly a worthy pursuit, but things get complicated when they try to translate these practices for the rest of us without romanticizing or appropriating the culture they come from. As I dove into learning about Ayurveda, I also wondered whether it was essential to learn Indian cooking in order to apply Ayurveda to one's life. I had this question for a while, and I worried whether it was somehow inappropriate, or that by asking it I would appear lazy. When I finally got up the courage to ask some Ayurvedic experts, I was relieved to learn that the answer is no, and that you can apply the process and principles of Ayurveda to just about any cuisine or culture and adapt it to fit your lifestyle.

Discovering Ayurveda's adaptability led me to a deeper understanding of this ancient tradition, and I'm happy to share the message far and wide. The beauty of these practices is that they exist in the process, and they're not exclusive to culture. Cooking and eating are as much about ritual as they are about the actual recipes and dishes that you are consuming. The food itself in Ayurveda is nourishing, but when we add the rituals of preparation, cooking, and eating at certain times of the day to support optimal health, we get the bigger picture. Your mind-set also matters. According to Ayurveda, food doesn't digest properly when you are experiencing grief, sorrow, or anger, or are getting too much or too little sleep.

Back in Illinois, lunch was the big, important meal of the day in my family, prepared by my grandma and my mom for my uncles when they came back from the farm for their midday break. Farmers head out before the sun comes up, and by noon they've already had a long day of work to recover from. This meal was fuel to keep them going for the rest of the day, but it was also about ritual. Refuge, rest, family, and nourishment were the essential ingredients, in addition to mashed potatoes, noodles, and a roast. This midday break gave them the rest they needed from an already long day of work and fortified them to go back to the fields until the sun set. It was also practical to break at noon, when the sun was at its highest and hottest.

Most of us aren't farmers, and we may not need the kind of hearty lunch that my uncles sat down to, but we can all cultivate our own rituals that support our lifestyles. We should understand that these rituals are as integral to health as the ingredients and the healing properties of the foods we ingest. If you are someone who often eats on the go, consider making the time to sit down and enjoy your meals. Rather than grabbing a sandwich for lunch and eating it in front of your computer at work, consider making it a ritual to eat at a communal table in a nearby café, or invite a coworker to eat with you. You'll give your body the time it needs to rest and digest, and you'll also enjoy the benefits of conversation.

The true meaning of Ayurveda is supporting optimal balance in your life through self-knowledge, food, and ritual. It's about slowing down and participating in the rhythm of life, instead of trying to be as busy as possible. It's about seeing the value in our lives in every moment, rather than pushing ourselves to the limit and only relaxing when we burn out. It's about learning what it means to nourish ourselves properly and to participate in the natural flow of life. That is what I hope to share with you, and I want you to keep this in mind as we embark on the reset portion of this chapter.

Okay, it's time for our reset to begin! As you journey through this section, try to stay grounded in the intentions we set at the start of this section, and let the system of Ayurveda be your guide without getting attached to dogma. You are doing this to improve your health and well-being, not for the purpose of becoming a servant to a system or a way of eating.

Eat Clean and Eat Well

Eating foods that are whole, fresh, and local is fantastic because sustainability aligns with a main principle of Ayurveda. Prana, the Ayurvedic term for life force, has to do with the energy you possess and the energy of what you consume. Foods rich in prana are those that come fresh, straight from the earth. Ayurveda teaches us that from the moment a food is picked, its prana begins to slowly fade. Eating as fresh as possible by shopping at local farmers' markets, or in the local section in your grocery store, or growing some of your own veggies supports your vital life force. If you've ever eaten an apple straight from the tree, or picked a raspberry and enjoyed it right away, you've experienced the extra-delicious taste and vibrance that eating fresh brings. This way of eating is so simple, but it gets confused because we have the modern convenience of being able to eat pretty much whatever we want, when we want it. Foods are shipped across the world and grown in greenhouses out of season, but these conveniences come at a cost both to the environment and to our health. We should shift our buying and eating habits to buy local and in season in order to support our vitality.

check in daily with how your feel

Once your 28-day *Clean Mind, Clean Body* detox ends, it is absolutely okay—and even healthy—to indulge occasionally in sweet treats and "fun foods" that break the Clean Eating Rules. But the key is moderation. You will still want to live by these guidelines, and fun indulgences should be the exception, not the rule. It's all about balance. The goal isn't restriction. It's satisfaction with who you are, and with how the way that you eat makes you feel.

Throughout Week 3, it's important to check in with yourself daily and to take stock of how you are feeling, both physically and emotionally. Are you are feeling deprived? Are you trying to override your cravings with force? If so, take the opportunity to reconnect with yourself and with your goals through one of the meditation exercises in chapter 1. When we are feeling stressed and out of balance mentally, we are more likely to reach for junk food or a processed treat and derail our goals. But we must keep sight of the fact that this is a quick fix, not something that will make us feel the way we want to feel long-term.

CLEAN EATING RULES

With all of that said, let's jump right into my Clean Eating Rules, which you are going to follow throughout Week 3, and which we should all aim to incorporate into the way we eat long-term.

Eating naturally and locally is great for you and it's great for our world. Venture to your local farmers' market and it's hard not to be inspired by the vibrant colors of the fresh fruits, veggies, homemade breads, and jams you will find there! It is of course possible to eat naturally and locally with foods from your neighborhood grocery store, too—just be sure to pay attention to what you're buying and where it was grown. This information is readily available, but we don't always pay attention to it.

The Environmental Working Group (EWG) is a trusted resource and activist group that reports on what is happening with produce, pesticides and GMOs, and our health. Check out their website, www.ewg.org, and read their reports to stay up to date on the food industry and topics like safe drinking water, public health, toxins, chemicals, consumer products, cosmetics, energy, and children's health. According to the EWG, pesticides have been linked to a variety of health problems, including brain and nervous system toxicity, cancer, and hormone disruption. The EWG publishes a list called "The Dirty Dozen" that tracks the produce items that contain the highest levels of pesticides, meaning that you are better off choosing organic versions of these fruits and veggies. It's great to buy all organic if possible, but when it's not an option or if you're eating on a budget, this is a nice resource to have.

THE DIRTY DOZEN

Strawberries	Apples
Spinach	Grapes
Kale	Peaches
Nectarines	Cherries

Pears	Potatoes
Tomatoes	Hot peppers
Celery	

The EWG also publishes a list called "The Clean Fifteen," the produce that contains the lowest amounts of pesticides, depending on the chemicals used in the crops and any other variables happening with the produce. This list, like The Dirty Dozen, is updated annually, so make sure to check EWG's website for the latest information. The EWG suggests that it's okay to choose conventional versions of these items, rather than organic, to spare your wallet.

THE CLEAN FIFTEEN

Avocados	Kiwis
Sweet corn	Cabbages
Pineapples	Cauliflower
Frozen sweet peas	Cantaloupes
Onions	Broccoli
Papayas	Mushrooms
Eggplants	Honeydew melons
Asparagus	

When I started paying more attention to choosing organic produce around fifteen years ago, I discovered that my shopping basket was suddenly full of more fruits and veggies and fewer packaged foods than I had previously been consuming. I wanted to have more energy, get sick less, and break the habit of relying on caffeine and sugar to keep me going. I started to pay attention to when local farmers' markets were happening, and at those farmers' markets, I discovered amazing locally grown foods and got to meet the growers themselves. There is magic in being more connected to what we consume. And if you think buying local and organic is more expensive, you might be surprised by the cash you can save by preparing foods with fresh produce instead of buying packaged or prepared foods. Michael Pollan, a go-to guru on this subject, tells us to shop only the periphery of the supermarket, because that's where the "real" food is (aka the produce, dairy, and meats). The middle aisles are to be avoided, because that's where you find the processed stuff, convenience foods that provide quick calories but don't do much for our health.

Meat and Dairy

Our global shift toward health consciousness and sustainability has made eating less meat and dairy, and even going vegan, part of a mainstream lifestyle. If you do choose to eat meat and dairy, it is much better for your health and for the environment to eat local, organic, and hormone-free, and to stay away from factory-farmed meat and dairy. According to Ayurveda, whether you should eat these items depends on your constitution and health needs, and is of course a personal decision based on your values or religious practice. It's also essential to consider what modern science has discovered about the health effects of consuming meat and dairy. *The China Study*, a book based on a twenty-year study conducted by the Chinese Academy of Preventive Medicine, Cornell University, and the University of Oxford in the UK, illustrates the link between the consumption of animal products (including dairy) and chronic illnesses like coronary heart disease, diabetes, breast cancer, prostate cancer, and bowel cancer.

Ayurveda recommends eating meat in moderation, not on a daily basis, and to include it occasionally at the midday meal to allow plenty of time for digestion. Eggs, according to Ayurveda, are heavy and hard to digest, but highly nutritious, and people with strong digestive powers can include them regularly in their diet.

Even through the rising popularity of nondairy milks and cheeses, Ayurveda maintains its stance on the benefits of milk, yogurt, and ghee. The recommendation is grass-fed, organic, and (if possible) raw milk and dairy. Scientific research tells us that raw milk products can harbor dangerous microorganisms that can cause serious health risks. It's important to consider the ancient guidance of Ayurveda through the lens of modern science and of course to keep your common sense in check and your healthcare provider in the loop about your diet and lifestyle.

It is possible that in the near future, experts who carry the torch for Ayurveda might update the recommendations based on modern science. Regardless, it is always preferable to consume whole, fresh, locally grown foods farmed without pesticides or added chemicals. It's interesting to consider that Ayurveda developed long before the existence of commercial-scale food production and factory farms. Today, we have to consider a whole new set of conveniences and factors that can lead us away from making healthy food choices. As Ayurveda suggests, *you* are the most essential ingredient to your own well-being. So think critically when making food choices, visit your doctor for regular checkups, and modify your diet as necessary to meet your individual needs.

Clean Eating Rule 2:
Beware of Food Trends

In the moment, it's easy to get sucked in, but we don't have to look back very far to be reminded of how claims of "healthy" food trends can play out. Remember olestra in the 1990s? If you need a reminder, olestra was a calorie-free fat substitute that was approved by the FDA in 1996 as a replacement for fats and oils in prepackaged snack foods like potato chips and Doritos. Sounds too good to be true, right? It was. Side effects led the FDA to add the following health-warning label to all olestra products: "This product contains olestra. Olestra may cause abdominal cramping and loose stools." No wonder the stuff eventually lost its popularity. I remember being in high school when this trend hit, trying these chips, and experiencing the severe abdominal cramping myself. Yuck.

Dubious trends abound today. Edible collagen, for example, is an expensive supplement that promises better skin, hair, and nails and can be added to smoothies and coffee in powder form or taken as a pill. There is scant evidence that this stuff works, and medical professionals are skeptical, given that the collagen powder breaks down in the digestive system before it can reach the skin to provide the purported benefits. But in spite of the lack of conclusive research, collagen remains a popular product.

And the supplement industry as a whole is booming, with pills, powders, and potions being marketed to customers attached to a variety of wellness promises—better sleep, antiaging, reduced anxiety, gut health, and fertility, among other claims. Yet the supplement industry was unregulated by the FDA until 2019, meaning that manufacturers could claim health benefits for their products without any sort of research or testing to back up those claims. As a result, millions of people out there are taking supplements that may have no health benefits at all, and that may even be harmful. So be wary, and be smart—always consult your doctor or a trusted health professional before taking a new supplement or trying any sort of trendy health product.

Clean Eating Rule 3:
Eat to Support Digestion and the Flow of Your Day

This rule is a principle of Ayurveda, and it's one that we see reflected in Mediterranean countries like Spain, where long lunches are taken, followed by an afternoon break. This not the typical America practice, but we would greatly benefit from following it.

In Ayurveda, breakfast is light, allowing the body to gain energy from nourishment but not be bogged down by digestion demands. Lunch is the heaviest meal, giving the body time to digest the meal properly over the rest of the day. Dinner is lighter than lunch, allowing the digestive system to rest while you sleep. My grandmother eats this way, as a habit from life on a working farm. At ninety, she wakes at four A.M. with the energy to sew her famous quilts, and has coffee and something light like toast with peanut butter for breakfast. She works on her quilts till noon, and when relatives sometimes come over for a big spread, everyone takes a break to socialize and rest. For lunch she sets out a variety of dishes like fruit salad, soup, a roast, bread, and mashed potatoes. She often takes a nap in the afternoon. Then it's back to work, and dinner at five or six P.M. is usually something light, like leftovers from lunch. My grandmother hasn't studied the principles of Ayurveda, but the timeline of her day and her eating and working habits are aligned with this ancient practice.

This way of eating follows the flow of the day, but many of us override this flow in order to accommodate our hectic schedules. It may not be realistic for many of us to rise with the sun and take a long, leisurely lunch in the middle of the day. But at the very least, we should avoid eating lunch at our desks or in front of the computer, and make lunch a real meal that satisfies us and won't leave us starving by dinnertime. We can also aim to begin winding down earlier in the evening, have a lighter dinner, and avoid late-night snacking so that we'll sleep better and wake up feeling more rested. We can all reap the benefits by tuning in to our body's needs and simplifying our lives accordingly.

on intermittent fasting

Intermittent fasting derives from Ayurveda, which recommends that we eat our largest meal at midday, avoid snacking, and only have something very light for dinner to give the digestive system a full rest. Intermittent fasting has also gotten recent support from modern science, and it has emerged as a big diet trend over the past few years. There is evidence that intermittent fasting promotes weight loss and cellular repair, decreases inflammation, and reduces the likelihood of developing certain diseases. The way it works is that between meals, as long as we don't snack, our insulin levels go down and our fat cells can then release their stored sugar as energy. This sugar stored in our cells would otherwise be brought into our fat cells by insulin, but the idea is that if we allow our insulin levels to drop far enough for long enough, we burn off our fat.

The least extreme version, known as "time-restricted feeding," involves eating on a 16:8 schedule, meaning that you eat only during an 8-hour window each day and fast for the other 16 hours (typically between dinner and breakfast) to give your body a break from digestion and allow your insulin levels to go down. There are a variety of much more extreme versions of intermittent fasting, none of which I would recommend trying without consulting your doctor. Anyone with a history of eating disorders, as well as pregnant women and nursing moms, should avoid intermittent fasting.

I practice a gentler, simplified version of intermittent fasting, which I would recommend to you as the version to try, if it works for your lifestyle: avoid snacking at night and plan your evening so that you eat dinner on the early side. I usually eat dinner between five and six P.M., and I avoid snacking in the evening after dinner. I find that this improves my sleep and leaves me feeling more energized in the morning. It has also reduced my sugar cravings dramatically throughout the day. I used to crave a big bowl of ice cream before bed; I'd have one, but then I'd have a hard time sleeping and wake up groggy and feeling bloated. My goal is not weight loss, but intermittent fasting has improved the quality of what I eat at mealtimes, and it has improved my energy levels in the morning. If weight loss is one of your health goals, intermittent fasting could be a great sustainable lifestyle change for you. But think of it as a decision for your health and well-being, to be undertaken moderately, and not as a quick-fix diet.

Spices are an amazing way to add flavor to your dishes, and they have some great healing benefits as well. Here are a few of my favorite spices to cook with.

Cinnamon—Balances blood sugar, contains antioxidants, is anti-inflammatory, and may lower the risk of heart disease. I love to grate it on baked apples, oatmeal, and rice dishes, or add a cinnamon stick to my tea.

Turmeric—Known for its antioxidant and anti-inflammatory properties, turmeric is the mother of well-being spices. Studies have shown that it protects and improves the health of virtually every organ in the body. Enjoy it in rice dishes, sprinkled over vegetables, in soups, and in salad dressings.

Ginger—Called universal medicine (*vishwabeshaja*) in Ayurveda, ginger is a healing staple with a kick. Ginger is known to boost circulation, fight off colds, and aid digestion. I love to add grated ginger to stir-fries, rice dishes, and soups, as well as to tea and smoothies.

Cumin—Used in many Mediterranean, Mexican, Middle Eastern, and Indian recipes, cumin has a plethora of benefits, including blood sugar and cholesterol control, and revving up digestion, and it is a good source of iron. Added to tea and drunk before bedtime, it's also great for sleep. Cumin can be easily added to soups, sauces, and salad dressings.

Coriander—Both the leaves of this plant (referred to as cilantro) and the seeds (referred to as coriander) can be used in cooking. It's a mild spice that can soothe an irritated digestive system. It's easy to incorporate into rice dishes, soups, baked veggie dishes, and salads.

Clean Eating Rule 5:
Cook for Yourself

Getting involved in the process of cooking is probably one of the best things you can do for your well-being. You don't have to be a top chef to get interested in preparing your own meals. Start with one meal a week—maybe it's dinner on Sunday—and see where that leads you. Cooking can be a great wellness practice, sparking creativity, reducing stress, and allowing you to slow down and reconnect with yourself.

My mom always teases me that I had no interest in cooking growing up and now it's a big part of my lifestyle. The shift for me began when I hit a breaking point with the stress in my life and wanted to feel better. I committed to shopping for more fresh produce and healthy grains, and I started asking friends for recipe recommendations, along with researching new recipes on my own. The key for me was simplifying these recipes as needed and swapping ingredients in and out to create my own unique versions that I loved. The freedom to start making recipes my own was what really got me excited about cooking.

In order to give yourself the freedom to improvise, it's important to have a good stock of staples in your kitchen. Beyond this, I recommend shopping for groceries weekly, depending on the specific meals you want to cook that week. Here is a list of my kitchen staples to aid you in your stocking up. When I have these items around, I can easily create a variety of meals for everyone, or something easy and quick just for myself.

SPICES

Cinnamon

Turmeric

Ginger (fresh and ground)

Sea salt

Black pepper

Red pepper flakes

Cumin

Coriander

PANTRY

Rolled oats

Basmati rice

Mung beans

Pasta

Rice noodles

Black beans

Cashews

Almonds

Peanut butter

Honey

Tea

Olive oil

Coconut oil

COUNTER

Apples

Bananas

Tomatoes

Potatoes

Fresh bread

FRIDGE

Oat milk

Leafy greens (in season)

Celery

Lemons

Limes

Mushrooms

Carrots

Broccoli

Yogurt (coconut)

Onions

Garlic

Clean Eating Rule 6:
Create Community Around Food

Eating together is encoded deep in our history and our cultural DNA, but we have allowed this practice to slip away in our busy modern lives, with many of us eating alone or eating on the go. Research from the University of Oxford reveals that the more often people eat with others, the more likely they are to feel happy and satisfied with their lives. People who eat socially are more likely to feel better about themselves and have a wider social network capable of providing social and emotional support.

Ayurveda reminds us that we need a healthy mind to be able to digest properly. There isn't a lot written about eating with community in Ayurvedic texts, likely because during the time of its origin, it was unimaginable that someone might be sitting at a desk or running to a meeting while eating. Breaking bread and sharing food with family, friends, and neighbors has been central to our survival as humans, both physically and socially. It's only in recent modern times that we have strayed from this commonsense well-being practice for the sake of our busy schedules. Eating every meal with others might be unrealistic, but it's great to aspire toward eating with others as much as possible as a wellness practice, and to prioritize it like we would our meditation and movement practices.

Clean Eating Rule 7:
Eat with the Season

Eating seasonally means eating food during the season in which it is naturally grown and harvested where you live. According to Ayurveda, eating seasonally helps us transition and thrive during each season of the year. Each season in Ayurveda corresponds to a dosha. During summer/pitta season, cooling foods like fresh fruits and salads are recommended. In the fall and early winter/vata season, warmer, more nourishing foods like soups, stews, and roasted root vegetables are recommended. For late winter and early spring/ kapha season, warm, cooked, slightly oily, and spicy foods are suggested.

Eating seasonally helps us align with nature and the rhythm

of the seasons. It also helps us connect to what is happening in the world around us, supports the local economy, and is better for the environment. Shopping at your local farmers' market or joining a local CSA (community supported agriculture) program is a great way to learn about what produce is harvested each season. Starting your own garden, whether in your yard, on your porch, or in a window box, is another way to learn about the growing process and enjoy the fruits (and herbs) of your labor. Even on a windowsill, you can plant and grow simple things like basil, mint, oregano, tomatoes, green beans, and salad greens. If growing your own fruits and vegetables seems intimidating, start with a fresh herb garden!

Meals and Recipes: Nourishment for the Whole Self

As a yoga instructor and former dancer, I have always relied on movement as the primary way that I stay connected to myself and improve my well-being. But the more time I spend exploring the healing power of food—not just through eating the food that I love, but by shopping for it or growing it, preparing it, and sharing it with others—the more I have come to understand that food is the main force in our overall well-being. It doesn't matter how much we meditate, practice yoga, and declutter our lives. If we have a fast-paced relationship to food, we aren't living well.

"Food is fuel" is a popular phrase, and a loaded one at that. If we only view food as fuel, we miss out on the way it truly nourishes and serves us. Some of us view cooking and spending time in the kitchen as unnecessary, or "not our thing," either because we think we're not interested or because we don't think we have the time. In my mind, that's like saying you don't have time to exercise or to take a shower. Cooking and eating well is an essential part of caring for our bodies!

With all this in mind, here are my favorite healing, nourishing recipes to help get your body, mind, and spirit in balance. The recipes featured here are all vegetarian and Ayurveda inspired, but feel free to add meat or a protein source like tofu if you like. I recommend that you eat "clean" during this detox period, meaning that you should eat whole, unprocessed foods, and organic as much as possible. I am not suggesting that you switch to an exclusively plant-based diet, unless that is something you are interested in exploring for your personal well-being, but it is widely acknowledged that there are health benefits to limiting meat and dairy. It's important to consult your healthcare professional when making a major diet change to account for your specific requirements. During Week 3 of your reset, try to swap these recipes in for some of your usual meals and snacks. And don't be afraid to make these recipes your own and improvise!

clean
body
recipes

turmeric latte

Drinking turmeric tea is one of the best ways to allow your body to make use of this healing root because of bioavailability, which means combining it with other ingredients in a way to make it more usable to your body. In this latte, combining turmeric with black pepper increases the bioavailability of the anti-inflammatory compound curcumin. The fat in the milk also aids absorption. Not to mention that this latte is delicious, fun to prepare, and a hit with guests who may show up expecting traditional tea or coffee. I make it in the afternoon, when I tend to hit a midday slump, and it gives me a much better boost than coffee!

You can use store-bought ground turmeric in this recipe, but I recommend buying whole fresh turmeric root, drying it out on a sunny windowsill for a few days or in a dehydrator or at a low temp in your oven, and then grinding it yourself in a food processor or high-powered blender. This is the best way to get fresh, super-charged ground turmeric and to stay in touch with the process of where your food comes from.

---

1 cup unsweetened oat milk or milk of your choice

½ cup filtered water

½ teaspoon ground cinnamon, plus more for garnish

½ teaspoon ground turmeric or DIY Turmeric Powder (recipe follows)

Pinch of ground black pepper

1 teaspoon ground ginger

1 teaspoon pure maple syrup

Homemade Coconut Whipped Cream (page 138), for serving (optional)

1. Whisk together the oat milk, water, cinnamon, turmeric, pepper, and ginger in a small saucepan. Bring to a gentle boil over medium heat. Reduce the heat to low and simmer for 10 minutes, then whisk in the maple syrup.

2. Remove from the heat, divide between two mugs, and sprinkle with cinnamon or top with coconut whipped cream.

DIY Turmeric Powder

5 or 6 (2- to 3-inch) pieces fresh turmeric root, peeled

1. Preheat the oven to 140°F. Place the turmeric on a baking sheet and bake for 5 hours, or until it is crispy. (Alternatively, place the turmeric on a plate on a sunny windowsill for a couple of days until the root has dried out.)

2. Transfer the dried turmeric to a food processor or high-powered blender and process into a powder. Sift the ground turmeric through a fine-mesh sieve to remove any larger chunks, if you like. Store in an airtight jar.

homemade coconut whipped cream

Coconut whipped cream is such a treat, and it's easier to make than you think! It's also so much better for you than the processed whipped cream that you probably grew up spraying from a can over desserts at every family gathering.

---

1 (13.5-ounce) can unsweetened full-fat coconut milk

1. Chill the unopened can of coconut milk in the fridge overnight.

2. Open the can and scoop the solid white cream from the top into a medium bowl. (Refrigerate the coconut water—the clearish liquid remaining in the can—for another use, such as a smoothie.)

3. Whip the coconut cream with a handheld mixer until peaks form.

4. Use immediately as a topping for your latte. Store any extra in an airtight container in the fridge for up to 3 days.

iced mint sun tea

As a former coffee addict, I know how challenging it can be to stay hydrated when you are constantly craving caffeine—which dehydrates the body! But if I can learn to strike a healthy caffeine balance, there is hope for anyone. Giving up caffeine cold turkey and only drinking water can feel extreme. This refreshing tea gives you a boost, while also nourishing and hydrating you. I learned this recipe from my mom, who used to make it in a giant glass jar out on our front porch in the summer. It can also be made inside close to a sunny window in the winter. Omit the green tea for a fully caffeine-free drink.

Filtered water

Large handful of fresh mint

1 teaspoon pure vanilla extract

1 tablespoon pure maple syrup (optional)

2 green tea bags (optional)

1. Fill a ½-gallon glass jar with water. Add the mint, vanilla, maple syrup (if using), and tea bags (if using).

2. Set the jar outside in the sun or near a sunny window and let stand for at least 1 hour, or until the water has changed color from clear to a greenish brown, depending on the exact type of mint and green tea you used. The longer you let the tea sit in the sun, the deeper the color will be and, if you used green tea, the stronger the drink will be.

3. Serve over ice, or blend each serving with a handful of ice for a delicious refresher.

agni tea

This tea is a staple in Ayurveda and will really get your digestive fires going. Make yourself a cup to enjoy first thing in the morning. For a pro move, you can even make a big batch to store in a thermos to drink throughout the day. You'll get hooked on the ritual of preparing this tea and how great it makes you feel!

---

4 cups filtered water
2 handfuls of sliced fresh ginger
2 teaspoons sea salt
1 teaspoon cayenne pepper
Juice of 1 lime

1. In a small saucepan, combine the water, ginger, salt, and cayenne and bring to a boil over medium heat. Boil for 20 minutes.

2. Remove from the heat and add the lime juice. Strain, let cool, and enjoy.

strawberry cooler

This berry-infused cooler is a great way to get your antioxidants in and to enjoy something just a bit sweet, satisfying, and refreshing. This drink is on repeat at our house for those afternoons when I need a pick-me-up and some good vibes.

---

1 cup fresh strawberries
1 cup ice
1 cup filtered water
Juice of ½ lime
Juice of ½ lemon
1 tablespoon pure maple syrup (optional)

Combine all the ingredients in a high-powered blender. Blend until smooth, pour into glasses, and chill out!

citrus cilantro creamy smoothie

With the cooling properties of citrus and cilantro, this healing and delicious smoothie is a great way to start your day or give yourself a midday pick-me-up. Add extra chili powder for a kick!

---

1 ripe banana (fresh or frozen), peeled

1 cup fresh cilantro

½ teaspoon chili powder

½ cup fresh orange juice

½ cup unsweetened oat milk

Combine all the ingredients in a high-powered blender. Blend until smooth, pour into glasses, and enjoy.

ooey-gooey protein smoothie

SERVES 2

This smoothie is perfect for a quick breakfast or as a midafternoon snack. It's great nourishment, and it feels like a luxurious indulgence.

---

1 tablespoon nut butter (almond, peanut, or cashew works great)

2 cups unsweetened almond milk or oat milk

4 dried dates, pitted

½ teaspoon pure vanilla extract

¼ teaspoon ground cinnamon

¼ teaspoon ground cardamom

Combine all the ingredients in a high-powered blender. Blend until smooth, pour into glasses, and enjoy!

turmeric ginger banana mango smoothie

SERVES 2

This delicious smoothie is a quick and easy way to boost your well-being with some superpowered turmeric. It's a great breakfast on the go or as a midafternoon pick-me-up snack.

1 ripe banana, peeled
½ cup fresh or frozen mango chunks
1 cup unsweetened almond milk or oat milk
½ teaspoon ground cinnamon
½ teaspoon ground turmeric
½ teaspoon fresh grated ginger

Combine all the ingredients in a high-powered blender. Blend until smooth, pour into glasses, and enjoy.

turmeric ginger banana mango nice cream

"Nice cream" is basically a frozen banana tossed in a high-powered blender and blitzed until it looks like ice cream. It's a great way to enjoy the deliciousness of ice cream without the bellyache that often comes from eating dairy. And with these special nourishing ingredients added, it becomes a must-have dessert! Turn your smoothie into "nice cream" with a few simple steps.

---

1 ripe banana, peeled and frozen

½ cup frozen mango chunks

½ teaspoon ground cinnamon

½ teaspoon ground turmeric

½ teaspoon fresh grated ginger

Combine all the ingredients in a high-powered blender. Blend until smooth, pour into bowls, and enjoy!

extra oat-y ginger cinnamon oatmeal

This recipe is so simple, and I include it here because starting the day with something that sticks to your stomach and warms your insides is essential.

½ cup rolled oats

1 cup filtered water

1 tablespoon chopped fresh ginger

1 teaspoon ground cinnamon, plus more for garnish

1 teaspoon ground cardamom

½ cup unsweetened oat milk

1 tablespoon peanut butter (optional)

1. Combine the oats, water, ginger, cinnamon, and cardamom in a medium saucepan over medium heat. Stir consistently until the water boils and the oats bubble a bit, about 5 minutes.

2. Add the oat milk and cook, stirring occasionally, for about 5 minutes more, until the oatmeal is thick and creamy. Remove from the heat.

3. Divide between two bowls and top with the peanut butter, if desired, or sprinkle with extra cinnamon.

baked cinnamon apple crumble

Great for a warming breakfast or a satisfying snack, this dish has the added bonus of making your kitchen smell fantastic. With the healing properties of ginger and cinnamon, it's the perfect combination of well-being and decadence in a bowl.

---

1 cup quick-cooking oats

1 cup oat flour

3 tablespoons butter or nondairy butter

¼ cup pure maple syrup

½ cup filtered water

1 tablespoon ground cinnamon

1 tablespoon sliced fresh ginger

6 apples, any variety, cored and chopped into 1-inch cubes

1. Preheat the oven to 350°F.

2. Combine the oats, flour, butter, maple syrup, water, cinnamon, and ginger in a medium bowl and mix with your hands to combine. Add the apples and mix to coat.

3. Pour the mixture into a 9 x 13-inch glass baking dish, cover with aluminum foil, and bake for 40 minutes, or until the apples start to fall apart. Enjoy warm.

banana mango salad with cilantro

An Ayurveda staple is banana with lemon and cilantro. It's fun to add whatever fresh fruit you have around to the mix. Mango is a great addition in the summer.

---

2 bananas, sliced

1 cup chopped fresh mango

½ cup fresh cilantro

1 teaspoon chili powder

½ teaspoon fresh lemon juice

Place all the ingredients in a medium bowl and toss to combine. Serve and enjoy.

everyday kitchari

SERVES 4

Kitchari is a staple Ayurvedic dish. The Hindi word *kitchari* means "mixture," and the dish itself is a mix of basmati rice and mung beans. Kitchari is easy on the digestive system and is believed to balance the doshas—think rice and beans with healing properties. My kitchari recipe, made with turmeric, cinnamon, ginger, oat milk, and a bit of maple syrup, is a simplified version of classic kitchari, which might include cloves, bay leaves, cardamom pods, fennel seeds, ground coriander, mustard seeds, cumin seeds, cilantro, and ghee.

You can also steam veggies like broccoli, carrots, and celery and serve them over your kitchari for a more robust meal. This dish keeps well in the fridge for several days and it's great for breakfast, lunch, or even as a cold snack.

---

1 cup dried split yellow mung beans (yellow mung dal)

1 cup uncooked basmati rice

2 tablespoons coconut oil or untoasted sesame oil

2 teaspoons ground turmeric

1 teaspoon grated fresh ginger

1 teaspoon ground cinnamon

1 teaspoon freshly ground black pepper

1 teaspoon sea salt

4 cups filtered water

1 cup unsweetened oat milk

2 tablespoons pure maple syrup (optional)

Fresh lemon juice (optional)

1. Rinse the beans and rice together in a strainer until the water runs clear.

2. Heat the coconut oil, turmeric, ginger, cinnamon, pepper, and salt in a medium saucepan over medium heat. Add the beans and rice along with the water. Cover and simmer over medium heat for 30 minutes.

3. Add the oat milk and simmer until the beans and rice are soft, about 10 minutes, stirring in the maple syrup during the last few minutes of cooking. Remove from the heat.

4. Divide the kitchari among four bowls and squeeze lemon juice over the top, if desired.

calm the vata veggie soup

Chicken soup doesn't have to be the only meal for the soul. As I've mentioned, it's important to eat with the seasons, and this recipe is perfect for doing just that. Calm the Vata Veggie Soup is meant to be adaptable, and this recipe can handle just about any seasonal veggie you might find at your local farmers' market. This version is made with broccoli and potatoes, but swap in whatever you like for either or both of these ingredients. Following this recipe is a list of additional seasonal veggies you could sub in.

2 tablespoons coconut oil
½ red onion, chopped
1 garlic clove, chopped
1 head broccoli (or vegetable of your choice), chopped
2 organic potatoes (or vegetable of your choice), chopped
1 teaspoon ground turmeric
1 teaspoon grated fresh ginger
A big pinch of freshly ground black pepper
1 teaspoon sea salt
Filtered water, as needed
1 cup unsweetened coconut milk or nondairy milk of your choice

1. Heat the coconut oil in a large saucepan over medium heat. Add the onion and garlic and sauté for 2 to 3 minutes, until softened, then stir in the broccoli, potatoes, turmeric, ginger, pepper, and salt.

2. Add water to the pot until the veggies are just barely covered. Bring to a boil, then reduce the heat to medium and simmer for 20 minutes, or until the veggies are soft.

3. Add the milk, stir, and raise the heat to high. Cook, stirring occasionally, for 3 to 4 minutes, until the milk is warm and combined well with the veggies. Remove from the heat.

4. If desired, carefully transfer the soup to a food processor and process to a puree, or serve as is. The soup keeps well in an airtight container in the refrigerator for up to 7 days.

spring veggies	summer veggies
Potatoes	Cauliflower
Mushrooms	Celery
Corn	Potatoes
Asparagus	Cabbage
Broccoli	Asparagus
Kale	Broccoli
Radishes	Collard greens
Onions	Beet greens
Chiles	Green beans

fall veggies	winter veggies
Beets	Eggplant
Carrots	Potatoes
Pumpkins	Beets
Squash	Carrots
Sweet potatoes	Spinach
Onions	Onions
Garlic	Corn
Okra	Mushrooms
Chiles	Winter squash

a-list asparagus soup

Asparagus makes the A-list in Ayurveda, as it suits all three doshas. Packed with nutritious minerals, it's also known for supporting reproductive health. Enjoy this alongside my Everyday Kitchari for a satisfying lunch, or on its own for a simple dinner.

---

1 tablespoon olive oil

1 garlic clove, chopped

2 cups asparagus (woody ends trimmed off), chopped

1 cup organic potatoes, chopped

1 cup filtered water

½ teaspoon Garam Masala Mix (see page 155) or store-bought

½ teaspoon sea salt

½ teaspoon freshly ground black pepper

1 cup unsweetened oat milk

1. Heat the olive oil in a medium saucepan over medium heat. Add the garlic and sauté until soft, about 5 minutes.

2. Add the asparagus, potatoes, water, garam masala, salt, and pepper. Bring to a boil, then reduce the heat to low, cover, and simmer for about 10 minutes. Add the oat milk and simmer for 5 minutes more. Remove from the heat.

3. Carefully transfer the soup to a high-powered blender, working in batches if necessary, and blend until smooth. Enjoy!

spicy creamy cauliflower and broccoli

Comfort food with a kick. It's incredible how creamy and satisfying this dish is, while skipping the tummy ache a giant bowl of mac and cheese can leave you with. Cauliflower and broccoli give this dish some major hearty vibes, but you can play around with substituting veggies you have on hand.

---

1 cup raw cashews, soaked for 15 minutes and drained
Juice of ½ lemon
¼ cup nutritional yeast
1 teaspoon ground turmeric
1 teaspoon red pepper flakes
½ cup unsweetened oat milk, almond milk, or filtered water
2 cups chopped cauliflower
1 cup chopped broccoli

1. Preheat the oven to 350°F.

2. Combine the cashews, lemon juice, nutritional yeast, turmeric, red pepper flakes, and oat milk in a high-powered blender. Blend until creamy.

3. Put the cauliflower and broccoli in a large bowl, pour over the cashew mixture, and toss to coat.

4. Transfer the mixture to a 9 x 13-inch glass baking dish and bake for 40 minutes, or until the edges of the cauliflower and broccoli are browned and crispy.

garlic chickpeas with spinach and tomato

SERVES 4

This warming, grounding dish is major comfort food with just the right combination of protein and veggies to leave you feeling nourished and satisfied. Perfect for a midday meal or for dinner.

3 tablespoons olive oil

5 garlic cloves, chopped

1 tablespoon chopped fresh ginger

2 cups sliced fresh tomatoes, such as cherry or Roma (plum) tomatoes

½ teaspoon red pepper flakes

½ teaspoon chopped fresh parsley

½ teaspoon fennel seeds

½ teaspoon sea salt

1 (15-ounce) can chickpeas, drained and rinsed

2 cups fresh spinach

Juice of 1 lime

¼ cup filtered water

1. Heat the olive oil in a medium saucepan over medium heat. When the oil is hot, add the garlic, ginger, tomatoes, red pepper flakes, parsley, fennel, and salt and simmer until the tomatoes start to fall apart, about 10 minutes.

2. Add the chickpeas and stir. Cook until they are lightly browned, about 10 minutes. Add the spinach, lime juice, and water and stir. Simmer until the spinach is wilted and everything is well mixed together, about 5 minutes. Remove from the heat.

3. Enjoy while hot.

turmeric ginger mashed potatoes

SERVES 2

Mashed potatoes are the ultimate comfort food, and a go-to side dish in our house. This Ayurveda-inspired twist includes turmeric and ginger, enhancing the warming and healing properties of the dish.

---

5 Yukon Gold potatoes, peeled

Filtered water, as needed

2 tablespoons olive oil

½ head garlic, chopped

1 tablespoon finely chopped fresh ginger

½ teaspoon ground turmeric

½ teaspoon sea salt, plus more as needed

½ teaspoon red pepper flakes

½ cup unsweetened oat milk

1. Place the potatoes in a medium saucepan and add water to cover. Salt the water, then bring to a boil over medium heat. Cook the potatoes until tender, then drain them and set aside.

2. Combine the olive oil, garlic, ginger, turmeric, salt, and red pepper flakes in a medium skillet and heat over medium heat, stirring consistently, until the garlic is soft, about 5 minutes. Remove from the heat and set aside.

3. Combine the potatoes, garlic mixture, and oat milk in a blender or in a large bowl and blend or beat with a handheld mixer until creamy.

magic masala rice and veggies

Garam masala is a spice mix used to season many traditional Indian dishes. In Hindi, *Garam* means "hot" and *masala* means "spice," and in Ayurveda, the mixture is thought to heat the body. You can buy premade garam masala in the spice section at your grocery store, you can grind your own spice blend, or you can do what I do and create your own mix from what you have in your spice rack. I like to add turmeric to my mix, which is not part of traditional garam masala, but the Ayurveda police haven't come knocking yet. Once you find a combination of spices you love, make a big batch and store it in a glass jar as a reminder of your goddess-like inspiration in the kitchen.

---

2 tablespoons coconut oil

2 garlic cloves, chopped

1 onion, chopped

2 organic potatoes, chopped

2 carrots, chopped

1 head broccoli, chopped

2 teaspoons Garam Masala Mix (recipe follows) or store-bought

2 cups Tomato Puree (recipe follows) or canned

½ cup filtered water

1 teaspoon red pepper flakes

½ cup coconut milk

Everyday Kitchari (page 147) or cooked basmati rice, for serving (optional)

1. Heat the coconut oil in a medium saucepan over medium heat. Add the garlic and onion and sauté for 2 to 3 minutes, until softened.

2. Stir in the potatoes, carrots, broccoli, red pepper flakes, and garam masala. Add the tomato puree and water and simmer for 20 minutes. Stir in the coconut milk and remove from the heat.

3. Serve as is, or with kitchari or basmati rice.

garam masala mix

1 teaspoon ground cumin
1 teaspoon ground coriander
1 teaspoon ground cardamom
1 teaspoon freshly ground black pepper
1 teaspoon ground cinnamon
1 teaspoon ground turmeric
½ teaspoon nutmeg, ground
½ teaspoon sea salt

Combine all the ingredients in a small jar and mix together well. Store away from light and heat and use within 6 to 12 months for best flavor.

tomato puree

MAKES ABOUT 2 CUPS

You can use canned tomato puree for the Magic Masala Rice and Veggies on page 154, but why not make your own? It's easy! Make a big batch and store any extra in the fridge for up to a week to use in soups and sauces.

Filtered water, as needed
2 or 3 Roma tomatoes

1. Bring a medium saucepan of water to a boil. Drop the tomatoes into the pot and boil for 5 minutes, or until their skins split.

2. Drain and peel the tomatoes. Cut the flesh into small pieces, transfer to a blender, and puree. Run the puree run through a sieve after blending to separate out the seeds. Store any unused puree in an airtight container in the refrigerator for up to 1 week.

crispy garlic healing potatoes

These crispy potatoes are super easy to make and as delicious and satisfying as your favorite fries, only healthier!

---

5 tablespoons olive oil

5 garlic cloves, chopped

1 teaspoon sea salt

2 cups Honey Gold potatoes or other small potatoes, halved

1 teaspoon ground turmeric

1. Heat the olive oil in a medium skillet over medium heat (the oil should thickly coat the pan). Add the garlic and salt and place the potatoes in the skillet cut-side down. Sprinkle the turmeric over the potatoes. Cook for 10 minutes, stirring occasionally, until the potatoes are browned.

2. Reduce the heat to low and cover the skillet with a lid. Cook for 20 minutes, or until the potatoes are very tender. Remove from the heat and enjoy!

fire it up tacos

These tacos add fun variety to your recipe repertoire. We love routine in our house, and whether we are at home for a long stretch, or traveling, I always try to make similar meals. These tacos are what I often call a "miracle meal": when you open the fridge and it seems like there's nothing left to pull something together, but from leftover veggies and some rice and tortillas, you make a miracle. The veggies included in this recipe are great, but feel free to improvise with what you have on hand to make your own miracle meal.

---

1 tablespoon coconut oil
½ onion, chopped
1 head cauliflower, cut into florets
2 garlic cloves, chopped
1 teaspoon red pepper flakes
1 teaspoon ground turmeric
½ teaspoon sea salt
1 cup cooked basmati rice
1 lime, halved
4 corn tortillas, for serving
1 avocado, chopped
Salsa or hot sauce, for serving

1. Combine the coconut oil and onion in a medium skillet and sauté over medium heat for 2 to 3 minutes, until the onion is softened.

2. Add the cauliflower florets, garlic, red pepper flakes, turmeric, and salt and sauté for 5 minutes, or until the cauliflower softens.

3. Add the cooked rice and squeeze the lime halves over the mixture. Cook, stirring, for 1 to 2 minutes. Remove from the heat.

4. Build your tacos on the tortillas, topping the cauliflower mixture with the avocado chunks. Serve with salsa or hot sauce.

coconut banana bread

SERVES 8

This healthy and delicious banana bread is perfect as a snack or for dessert. And this is a great way to use up all the ripe (or overripe) bananas in your kitchen. This recipe is a favorite in our house for its natural sweetness.

3 tablespoons butter or nondairy butter, melted, plus more for greasing

3 ripe bananas, peeled

1 large egg or equivalent egg substitute

½ cup coconut yogurt

2 cups oat flour

1 teaspoon baking powder

1 teaspoon baking soda

1 teaspoon ground cinnamon

½ teaspoon sea salt

1. Preheat the oven to 350°F. Grease a 9 x 13-inch glass baking dish with butter.

2. Mash the bananas in a large bowl. Stir in the melted butter, egg, and yogurt. Sift together the flour, baking powder, baking soda, cinnamon, and salt into a separate bowl, then add the dry ingredients to the bowl with the wet ingredients and stir to combine.

3. Pour the batter into the prepared baking dish. Bake for 50 minutes, or until a fork inserted into the center comes out clean.

4. Let the banana bread cool in the baking dish for 10 minutes, then turn it out onto a wire rack to cool completely before serving.

calming apple rice pudding

SERVES 2

This comforting dish is a nice way to wind down after a stressful day, with just the right amount of healing properties. I also like it as a midday snack for a pick-me-up.

½ cup uncooked basmati rice, soaked for 1 hour and drained

2 apples, cored and finely chopped

¼ cup raisins

1 cup unsweetened oat milk or almond milk

½ teaspoon ground cinnamon

½ teaspoon pure vanilla extract

Combine all the ingredients in a medium saucepan and cover with the lid ajar so steam can escape. Cook over medium-low heat, stirring occasionally, for 30 minutes, or until creamy.

Be in Your Body

This portion of our journey is also an opportunity for you to get back in touch with what it feels like to "be in your body." What I mean by that is, I want you to try to remember a time when you had a great relationship with your body and the way that nourishing it made you feel. This may be more challenging for some of us than for others. Maybe it was when you were five, maybe it was when you were a teenager, or maybe it was even more recently. Think back to this connection and focus on how great and free it felt. Your body felt strong and capable and you used it to enjoy life. You ate what felt nourishing and delicious to you. You ate intuitively and without worry or guilt about whether you were eating too much or too little, good stuff or bad stuff. If you can't recall a time in the past where you felt this connection between the way you were eating and the way you felt in your body, I'm incredibly excited for you. Because you *can* have this experience by embracing these practices.

As you approach the end of Week 3, I want you to ask yourself the questions that follow, which are modified versions of the questions that you asked yourself at the start of the chapter. Write down what comes up for you and compare your answers to where you were when you started Week 3. Reflect on whether this new way of eating feels like a more sustainable way of living and relating to food for you.

- How do you feel when you wake up in the morning? How does your diet contribute to this feeling?

- How has it felt to take the time to cook and enjoy real meals, as opposed to eating on the go?

- Do you experience anxiety surrounding food? Does thinking about what you will eat make you worried or stressed?

- Are grocery shopping and cooking a joy or are they dreaded tasks? Do you enjoy preparing meals?

- How has it felt to eat your meals with others while engaged in conversation and the act of eating?

- Do you still experience the same cravings for stimulating foods like sugar and caffeine to keep you going throughout the day, or foods with a particular taste or texture (salty, crunchy, etc.)? How has this changed?

- Do you still experience cravings at particular times of the day?

- At times when you weren't feeling great mentally or physically, how did that affect your food choices?

Be compassionate with yourself in your answers and know that nourishing your body is a constant process, forever changing as your body's needs change. Every moment is an opportunity to make a choice that better serves you.

People Who Are Living It Right

I want to introduce you to two women I admire immensely who are amazing at nourishing themselves not only with food, but with a life pointed toward balance. These friends of mine manage to juggle successful careers while maintaining their true well-being by caring for their bodies and eating well, first and foremost. I hope you are as inspired by these ladies as I am and motivated to forge your own path toward radiant nourishment and well-being.

JASMINE HEMSLEY
on Living the Ayurvedic Life with Ease

Jasmine is a bestselling author, chef, and Ayurvedic expert. She is always on the go, lending her recipes to top restaurants, giving lectures, and hosting wellness retreats. At the same time, she really practices what she preaches, in terms of taking the time to slow down and nourish her body while maintaining a busy schedule.

You are known for bringing Ayurveda to a mass audience. What do you see as the biggest challenges for someone wanting to integrate Ayurveda into daily life?

A big challenge we face is that modern life and technology cut us off from the flow of nature. This makes it difficult to tune in to the natural cues surrounding us—for example, the fading light of sunset that prompts melatonin production in our bodies, making us want to wind down for healing sleep. The blue light we're constantly absorbing from screens, as well as public lighting, disrupts and overrides this most natural of processes. Instead, we get home from work and watch TV or scroll through social media, and that all-too-familiar wired feeling occurs even when we're exhausted and should be going to bed.

Ayurveda gives us the tools we need to stick closer to nature and gently maintain the natural balance and harmony of mind, body, and spirit. It serves as a helping hand to allow us to thrive, but we can feel self-conscious about using these tools when the society we live in doesn't support a holistic approach to life. For example, I've been on jobs where someone has announced, "I'm taking ten minutes out to meditate," and others either nod their approval and carry on or join in! Then that person comes back refreshed and ready to get back to work. But for many people, the idea of breaking to meditate or to have a proper lunch during the workday is almost unimaginable! Luckily, there's an incredible resurgence of people looking to care for themselves in a more holistic way, and this is helping to change perceptions.

Is there a most-healing ingredient that everyone should have in their kitchen?

In Ayurveda, digestive health is key to your overall well-being, from how well you can utilize the food that becomes you to how well you can digest life's experiences. With that in mind, mung dal is the key ingredient in my kitchen (alongside my spice tin!). Mung dal is a tiny yellow pulse (not to be confused with other yellow lentils), the split and hulled version of whole mung beans (the little guys in the green jacket with a white flash). I always have it on hand, especially to make one of my most go-to, most delicious, and most comforting dishes: kitchari. Kitchari is a classic Ayurvedic dish that's well-balanced, easily digestible, versatile, and suitable for everyone—a melting pot of mung dal and basmati rice with plenty of spices (all of which have their own distinctive healing properties). Mung dal is protein-rich, making it wonderful for vegans, as well as being economical, easy to cook (it doesn't require soaking and takes less time to cook than other types of legumes), and easy to digest. In Ayurveda, it's known as tridoshic (meaning it will agree with almost anyone's mind-body constitution) and *sattvic* (meaning it is a harmonious, balancing food).

How do you accommodate Ayurveda in a busy lifestyle, especially when you're on the go and it's a challenge to cook all your meals?

Ayurveda is a philosophy, an understanding of nature that is designed to make life an easier ride for us. In this busy modern world, it's not realistic to expect to do everything "optimally," Ayurvedically speaking. But Ayurveda isn't meant to be black and white, just as nature ebbs and flows and can't be put into neat little boxes. There is always a better choice or even choices you can make in any situation!

One thing that's nonnegotiable in my routine is taking a lunch break, however busy I am. If I don't, the alternative will lead to indigestion. When I'm busy, I'll use my slow cooker to make hydrating, one-pot meals like soups and stews, and I'll cook in bulk, so that I can pop leftovers into my thermos for a hot, ready-to-go meal. If I'm not home or I'm short on time, I'll apply Ayurvedic principles to the food that's available, prioritizing well-cooked, seasonal, organic foods over foods that are raw or served cold. I also eat slowly and mindfully, being grateful for the food that I have and thoroughly enjoying it where possible!

In Ayurveda, agni is really the number one thing to be concerned about, rather than focusing on what food suits which dosha. If you're sitting down to a meal with friends and family and you're not feeling the "burn" of hunger, you need to fire up that agni. Otherwise, you're dumping the fuel of a meal onto a low-burning digestive fire, which explains why some of the "healthiest" dishes don't digest well, while the "unhealthy" ones go down easy after a power hike or a good swim that fires up your need to refuel! To light this digestive fire, I'll have one of my ginger anise chews from my cookbook *East by West* before a meal, I'll nibble some fresh ginger, or I'll squeeze half a lime into a small glass of water (you don't want to drink too much before or during a meal) and add a tiny pinch of salt. Within 10 to 15 minutes, you'll be salivating—if not before!

How do you integrate Ayurveda into your morning routine?

In oh-so-many ways! Ayurveda offers me a helping hand from the moment I wake up. The first thing I do in the morning is scrape my tongue with my Tongue Tingler, a simple practice that takes a few seconds and that helps clear the buildup that accumulates on the tongue overnight, in addition to preventing bad breath and helping to prevent infections. After that, I do 15 to 20 minutes of oil pulling while I'm in the shower to draw out impurities. I also do sun salutations and Vedic meditation in the morning, two pillars of the Ayurvedic lifestyle that get me in the mind-body space I need to go more mindfully about my day. Then I have a warming Ayurvedic breakfast like stewed apples, amaranth porridge, or—yep!—kitchari.

What is one simple thing we can do right now to get started with Ayurveda?

Eating your main meal at lunchtime between noon and two P.M., when your digestive fire, or agni, is at its strongest, is an easy way to do this, and it will truly energize you. Maintaining a healthy agni is key to feeling your best, as digestive problems in turn lead to general sluggishness, feeling run down, illness, and having to run to the toilet all the time—or perhaps not going enough! When you eat a well-balanced, easy-to-digest lunch, you leave the table feeling satisfied rather than overly full or with your mind still searching out flavors and textures. You'll naturally snack less, and the idea of eating an early, lighter, and easy-to-digest meal for supper will be more appealing, which is ideal for your digestion and will help you sleep more soundly. In turn, this will allow your body to focus on what it does best: healing and detoxifying, rather than processing that late-night steak. Such a simple switch in your eating habits can really enhance your life . . . as it did mine.

DR. ROBIN BERZIN
on Healing Foods and the Most Important Things We Can Do to Boost Our Well-Being

Dr. Robin Berzin is radicalizing healthcare and bringing functional medicine mainstream through her company, Parsley Health. She divides her time between the various branches of her office, serving local communities, and leading her team of doctors. Her knowledge of well-being and foods that heal is extensive, and she uses this knowledge to treat her patients and to nourish her own body as well.

What foods do you turn to for their healing properties?

I have a set of essential superfoods I keep in my life on loop, because when I'm steady with my diet I feel good. These foods include pasture-raised eggs (nature's B vitamin!), dark leafy greens and cruciferous veggies like kale and Brussels sprouts, raw organic almonds, extra-virgin olive oil (worth a splurge for the good stuff), wild salmon, and, for snacks, organic popcorn and kombucha.

In your medical practice, is there a superfood you recommend frequently to your patients?

In my book, the key to health is what you don't eat—refined flours, refined sugar, and processed foods. Avoiding these foods for the most part is 80 percent of eating well. Eating real, whole foods, most of which you cook yourself, is what makes food "medicine." Of course, we all love a slice of pizza, and I will indulge with my favorite vegan ice cream occasionally, but if you make 80 to 90 percent of your diet unrefined and unprocessed, then you can get away with eating the sugar and the flour here and there and not worry about it too much.

What are common ailments that people come to you for in your medical practice, and what lifestyle changes do you recommend to help?

We see men, women, and kids who have health issues across the board. This means GI issues (reflux, Crohn's disease, constipation, bloating); mental health issues (anxiety, depression, fatigue); heart health and blood sugar problems (from high cholesterol and blood pressure to metabolic syndrome and diabetes); autoimmune conditions (everything from eczema to multiple sclerosis); and hormone imbalances (think PMS, PCOS, infertility, menopause, and men's hormone issues).

So while it's really varied, we look at the whole person to start, and assess the history of what got them to this point. Often these problems started long ago, and understanding their origins can be really powerful for devising a treatment plan. From there, nutrition is always the starting place. Many people have food allergies and sensitivities they don't realize. For example, a patient of mine with nut allergies and seasonal allergies didn't realize he was also allergic to gluten and dairy—when he cut them out, his nut allergy and his spring seasonal allergies went away because he healed the inflammation in his system.

Other people are dependent on the up and down of a high-sugar, high-caffeine diet balanced with regular alcohol consumption that then leads to everything from fatigue, headaches, and weight gain to poor sleep and even depression and autoimmune conditions. For some people, starting there and eliminating these foods can be game-changing.

Do you have any tricks for keeping your energy up during the day, especially during the afternoon slump?

Yes! After an early dinner the night before, so you are able to intermittent fast, start your day with a high-healthy-fat, nutrient-dense breakfast like eggs and avocado. How you start the day will impact how you feel hours later. Second, when lunch comes, avoid carbs, which tend to give you a big up, then a big down around three P.M. Instead, for lunch, focus on cooked veggies, nuts and seeds, and sustainably raised/sourced protein. If you eat a salad for lunch, make sure that it has extra things like nuts and seeds and/ or a source of protein on it. I see a lot of people who eat a bowl of leaves for lunch and wonder why they are starving at three P.M. Third, drink plenty of water—sometimes that foggy feeling is actually dehydration, especially if you have had a coffee or two in the morning and that coffee is wearing off. Fourth, remember that coffee stays in your system for hours after you drink it. If you have it too late in the day—even after ten A.M.—it could be keeping you up at night and leading to poor sleep, which makes you even more tired and hungry the next day.

What is the most important thing we can do to improve our well-being?

There are two things! First, change the way you eat—cutting out refined sugars and flour and processed, packaged foods is a game-changer, as I mentioned earlier. From there, find some way to move your body, every day, that feels good. If going to a gym feels like a chore, find something else. Walking, yoga, weights, a team sport, dancing—whatever you like. When you move your body, you detox, stimulating positive endorphins that boost mood, as well stimulating insulin sensitivity, which keeps your blood sugar balanced. Exercise keeps your digestion moving—people forget that sitting a lot leads to a stopped-up gut. So find a form of exercise that you love to do and want to do for life. Or at least for now!

4

hit the reset:

change the way you move

It's not what happens to you, it's how you react to it that matters.
—Epictetus

Nowhere is the mind-body connection more relevant than in our relationship to physical exercise. There is abundant evidence showing us that our physical bodies are a reflection of our state of mind. Let's take stress and its effect on our bodies, for example. When we experience significant levels of stress, our bodies respond by producing a cascade of stress hormones that flood our systems. This stress response evolved in humans so that we could summon the strength to react quickly when in danger. Our modern problem is that we are continually activating this stress response with the unmanageable levels of stress in our lives, making our bodies think we are in intense danger all the time. Constant activation of this stress response takes a major toll on our bodies, contributing to high blood pressure, promoting artery-clogging deposits, and causing brain changes that may contribute to depression, anxiety, and addiction. High levels of stress have also been linked to decreased immunity, causing us to get sick more often, as well as to the tendency to put on extra weight.

Physical exercise is a great way to manage and reduce stress, strengthen our bodies, and keep us feeling healthy, energized, and balanced throughout the day—but only if that exercise is done with a calm mind. When we bring our stressed-out mind-set into how we approach exercise, we are inviting those stress hormones to make a home in us. We might say we feel better after a grueling workout, but that feeling is a bit of a mind trick. We feel better because the workout is over, but we have survived a mini trauma in the process. This is completely different from the experience of a workout that relieves stress and releases endorphins, leaving you feeling better about yourself.

I love talking with groups about this experience of a stressful workout versus one that relieves stress. After a stressful workout, people usually report that they are glad the workout is over and are more likely to want to "treat" themselves with an unhealthy meal that they have earned as a reward. The exhausting calculation of calories burned versus calories counted is perpetuated, and the endless cycle of punishment and reward is reinforced. In the opposite universe of a stress-relieving workout, people usually report feeling more in tune with themselves. They notice they want to continue that good feeling either by cooking for themselves or by spending time doing something mindful, creative, or productive. Your workout itself might only last for an hour or so, but it has long-term effects that shape and reinforce your habits.

Your workout routine may be guiding you toward a more calm, balanced, connected life, or pointing you toward more stress, tension, and destructive bad habits. It's important to pay attention to how your workouts are making you feel. If you tend to finish a workout feeling more stressed or exhausted than when you started, it may be time to consider making a change.

Some Personal Lessons on Mind-Set and Achieving

A few years ago I attended a CrossFit class as a part of a project I was working on for Reebok. CrossFit is the last place I would volunteer to be. I'm not practiced at lifting weights, and aggressive sports aren't something I gravitate toward. Before the class started, I asked the coach for any suggestions he had for me and what goal I should keep in mind. He was very nice and encouraging and told me the goal is to do as many repetitions as possible of each station before moving on to the next one. I was honestly relieved to know the goal was efficiency, although that isn't super obvious from an outsider's view. The goal we all see with something as intense as CrossFit is how heavy, how hard, how big you can go.

When the class began, I had the mind-set of having fun and doing my best to achieve the goal of as many repetitions as possible per station. I found that I enjoyed the aspect of CrossFit where everyone does the exercises together, and I let this feed my positive mind-set. One of the early stations was "wall balls," where you do a squat holding a medicine ball, come up to stand as you throw the ball against the wall, catch it, squat back down, and repeat. We were counting our squats. After the whistle was blown, signaling that we should move to the next station, I noticed I made it to the next station before all of my classmates. I'm not more experienced, better, faster, or stronger, but I have spent a lot of time practicing moving in the best way possible for my body, as well as being good to myself in that process. When the whistle was blown, I squatted down, released the ball quickly and gently, and headed efficiently over to the next station, wasting no energy. My classmates had a different approach to changing stations. They slammed the ball down with an added yell for maximum calorie-burning effect and stomped over to the next station with a power-through attitude. Our choreography was very different.

My speed between all the stations stood out over the class and I finished with a smile. I excelled in transitions, even though they were not a focus of the class. For me, the opportunity was in how we get everywhere we are going. The class was very challenging. I could have worn myself out even more by going to the next station with as much tension as possible, but instead I chose to make each transition with as much ease and efficiency as possible. I don't think being a CrossFit world champion is in my future, but I accomplished a higher number of repetitions that anyone thought would be possible for me, mainly because I crushed the transitions, and I had a lot of fun in the process.

I had a similar experience with an all-women's Spartan Race that I participated in (also for a partnership with Reebok). The race involved challenging obstacles like swimming through a natural lake, crawling under barbed wire, and lots of wall climbing. I did the race with a group of friends, and I honestly had fun the whole time. My teammates were accomplished obstacle-race athletes, and I was brand-new. I was pleased that I didn't hold them back at all and walked away injury-free. The difference again was in my mind-set of deciding to enjoy myself and also find the most efficient way for my body to accomplish each task.

There was one particular obstacle that stands out to me. We were given a heavy sandbag and asked to drag it up a steep hill and back down. All the women around me in the race dragged the heavy bag on the ground, which was quite taxing for their backs, but they could do it because they were all very strong, much stronger than me. These women would stop and take short breaks up the steep hill to let the pain subside and to psych themselves up. My first thought upon seeing this challenge was that there was no way I would be able to drag that heavy bag up that hill like those strong women, and that I didn't want to hurt my back trying. Instead of giving up, I found a better way for me. I hiked the bag over my shoulders, put a bend in my knees, and leaned forward slightly to even out. Balancing the bag over my shoulders was manageable for me. I ran up the hill and jogged down with a smile. I was proud of myself for trying to find a better way, and succeeding. Similar to my CrossFit class, I don't think I will be training to win any obstacle races anytime soon, but I have an approach to accomplish hard things in the best way for my body. It's great when your approach in one area of life works for many areas of life.

Exercise Doesn't Have to Hurt

I'm not a bodybuilder or an endurance athlete, which is probably pretty clear if you have read this far. I wanted to share these stories with you to show how it's possible to overcome challenging physical situations by choosing to find a better way to move and committing to a positive mind-set, rather than relying on force and aggression to get through the task.

I don't believe that exercise should involve physical suffering. Finding the most efficient way to move your body is the best way to accomplish more. When we believe suffering is our best path to accomplishment, we limit ourselves dramatically. We are so used to identifying pain as a sign of success that we get used to feeling unwell and performing sub-optimally. Shifting our mind-set to one of positivity and self-empowerment when it comes to exercise is our first step. Changing how we move is the next. Together, these two shifts are a winning combination for physical wellness and balance.

I'm rarely the strongest or fastest person in a room, but I'm committed to using my body as efficiently and harmoniously as I can during physical activity, and to enjoying the process. I practice ease and efficiency of movement whether I'm doing yoga, playing with Daisy, or in a high-intensity situation like a CrossFit class or Spartan Race. My goal isn't to be the better than someone else—it's to do what's possible for me. My goal is to stay in the process of a positive mind-set and efficient movement so I can reach my potential in all I do and enjoy every moment along the way. I know that when I stay in this process, I achieve more, feel more present, and experience gratitude for my life. This is what I want more of, and I know I'm not alone in wanting a life of achieving more, feeling better, and experiencing gratitude. There is a formula, but it's not in the workouts or the yoga. The magic is in you.

Body Positivity Made Real

Whether your preferred form of exercise is yoga or running, Spinning or lifting weights, if you are doing these physical activities without a clean mind, with negative self-talk or work stress running through your head, you are creating tension in your body, and the exercise may actually have adverse effects, including increasing muscle tension, hindering progress, making it harder to lose weight, and leading to a wide variety of digestive issues.

We are living in the era of "body positivity," which on the surface sounds great. But let's be sure that we aren't using this popular term as a mask, while anxiety, social media–induced body shame, and stress about the way that we look linger below the surface. In order to achieve true body love and acceptance, we must accept that our physical bodies are an expression of our mental and spiritual state, and the choices we make. Our bodies are capable of incredible things if we treat them well. They are our homes for life. So let's commit to making better choices for our bodies. Let's stop judging and objectifying, and start honoring our bodies with movement. And let's make this a daily practice.

be your own cheerleader

Your relationship with exercise is a continually evolving practice, and it begins in your mind. If you find yourself slipping into negative thought patterns during exercise, have patience with yourself, just as you do when your mind wanders during meditation. Remember that negative thoughts will sometimes drift in during exercise. Acknowledge them, and then gently return to your focus. When I feel the negative thoughts creeping in during exercise, I offer up the following prayer of love for my body. You may wish to borrow this prayer if it resonates with you, or come up with one of your own. The goal here is to encourage positive self-dialogue during physical exercise.

I am grateful for my body and the ways that it serves me.

I respect my body and will allow it to grow and change.

I love my body and will nourish it with healing movement.

I enjoy my body and will celebrate all that it allows me to do.

journal it out:
feel-good body goals

Now let's clear a path for the new relationship you are going to have with your body and with exercise. We're going to set some goals to this end, beginning with a series of questions. Jot down your responses as you reflect on these questions. We will come back to them again at the end of this chapter.

- How many times a week do you currently engage in structured exercise, like practicing yoga, going for a hike, or taking an exercise class? How many times a week would you ideally like to be able to exercise?
- During exercise, what is happening in your mind? Are you carrying mental stress and negativity with you into your workout?
- What kinds of exercise do you currently do, and what new kinds of exercise would you be open to trying?
- Do you tend to stay moving throughout your day, or do you spend most of your time sedentary?
- Are there opportunities throughout your day where you could incorporate more movement? Could you take the stairs instead of the elevator? Could you get up from your desk at work to take a walk? Instead of scrolling on your phone during your downtime, could you do a few planks or some stretching?

Based on your answers to these questions, what are some changes that you would like to make, in terms of your relationship with your body and with exercise? These are your Feel-Good Body Goals. Jot these down as well. As an example, here are my Feel-Good Body Goals:

- I want to practice yoga daily, even if just for 10 or 20 minutes.
- I want to challenge myself physically with a new exercise at least once a week.
- I want to exercise outdoors more, going for brisk walks and hikes.
- I want to take more breaks during my workday to do simple exercises, like planks.
- I want to feel good about my body and reflect regularly on my mind-set.

Now that you have established these goals as your guideposts for this chapter, let's get started. As with the previous chapters, there are the three phases we'll explore during Week 4 of your *Clean Mind, Clean Body* journey:

Moving Well: We'll practice getting into the flow, getting our mind-set right, and moving in harmony during ordinary movements we do each day.

Redefining Exercise: We'll change our habits with movement and create opportunities during our day to exercise and move well.

Getting Outside: When in doubt, go outside. We'll explore the healing power of the great outdoors. Whether you live in a city, in a suburb, or in the country, you can benefit from time spent in nature.

Moving Well

Don't force it! In our modern lives, many of us have come to believe that more always equals more, that maximum effort equals maximum return, in exercise and in life in general. We've convinced ourselves that if we aren't stressed out, both mentally and physically, we aren't working hard enough. But the truth is the opposite, particularly when it comes to the way we are moving our bodies. For example, if you feel anxious about making it to your cardio boot camp class, and end up clenching your jaw and tensing your forehead on the way there, you're creating more tension in your body and mind even though you are trying to do something good for yourself. If you beat yourself up mentally during a yoga class for not being strong or flexible enough, the practice doesn't have a chance to benefit you. When you find yourself tensing your body when you are mentally challenged at work, this also sets you off-balance.

It's important to recognize that these experiences are common to all of us. We all hold tension in our bodies, and this affects the way we move and function throughout the day. But when we take the time to notice habits that aren't serving us, we can make an effort to change and form new, better habits. Balance isn't a destination where you arrive, and suddenly things are perfect. Living in balance is a constant practice of noticing and making adjustments in order to feel better and more like yourself.

We have been told that sickness, burnout, tension, and stress are par for the course in our busy lives. These things have become our badges of honor, signs that we are working hard and getting the most out of life. But the truth is that these are warning signals, red flags that our body is raising, telling us to stop! Instead of pushing ourselves physically to the breaking point and forcing our bodies to do more than they want to do, we need to embrace a philosophy of efficient movement, the philosophy of "moving well," as I call it. We must move well in order to heal and restore our bodies, rather than wearing ourselves out, breaking ourselves down, or exhausting ourselves physically. When we move well, we discover our true potential, we can do more than we thought was possible, we have access to strength when we need it, and we are able to restore ourselves in the process.

When we push ourselves to the point of pain, whether going for a run or carrying out an everyday task like putting away groceries, we are not doing what's best for our bodies. Instead, we need to learn to move our bodies as efficiently as possible, and in a healthy range that allows old bad habits to dissolve and healthy ones that build whole-body strength to emerge. We can form a healthy relationship to challenges by practicing moving well. We can return to a more natural state of enjoying physical activity, rather than thinking of it as a chore or punishment.

Throughout this phase of Week 4, we are going to focus on moving harmoniously throughout our daily tasks, rather than thinking of physical activity as a necessary evil to be forced. We'll practice "moving well" in everyday movements, like waking up, putting away groceries, and walking in a more efficient way. It might seem silly to practice moving well when opening a door, standing, or making coffee, but we can't expect to move well during our structured workouts if we don't practice moving well in our everyday activities.

modern tai chi

When we think of tai chi, most of us conjure up images of older Chinese people practicing gentle, flowing exercises together in the park. But the overall philosophy includes so much more than a stress-reducing physical exercise. Tai chi is a way of life that has been practiced by the Chinese for thousands of years, passed on from generation to generation. Initially tai chi developed as a philosophy, and then evolved into a martial art, so the exercises that we recognize as tai chi today are only a few hundred years old. *Tai chi* means "the ultimate," and the practice involves improving and progressing toward the unlimited, the immense existence, and the great eternal. A guiding principle of tai chi is the theory of opposites: yin and yang, the negative and the positive. According to tai chi, the abilities of the human body are capable of being developed beyond our preconceived potential. Civilization can be improved to the highest levels of achievement. Creativity has no limit, and the human mind should have no restrictions on its capabilities. According to tai chi theory, one develops in the direction of this ultimate by balancing their natural yin and yang energy and moving in harmony with the self and with nature.

We can apply the vast and ancient wisdom of tai chi in ways that are practical for our modern lives. Tai chi emphasizes that our goals should be achieved through moderate, natural ways of living. And at the core of tai chi is the idea that we must work toward harmony of mind and body while staying in tune with nature. We create harmony in our lives starting with how we think (meditation), move (practice), and act (kindness and service). When we align how we move with grace and efficiency, we get into the tai chi flow and experience creativity, fulfillment, and well-being. Think of tai chi as a universal truth that exists inside of you, waiting to be discovered. This practice is a part of you already, and the joy is in claiming it.

MORNING PRACTICE FOR MOVEMENT: TAI CHI WAKE AND SHAKE

Here is a practice to add to your morning routine to energize your body upon waking and encourage harmonious movement throughout your day.

1. Roll out of bed and come to standing. Shift your hips from side to side to find the perfect wide, comfortable, and stable stance for your feet. Soften your knees a bit so you are moveable. Relax your arms by your sides.

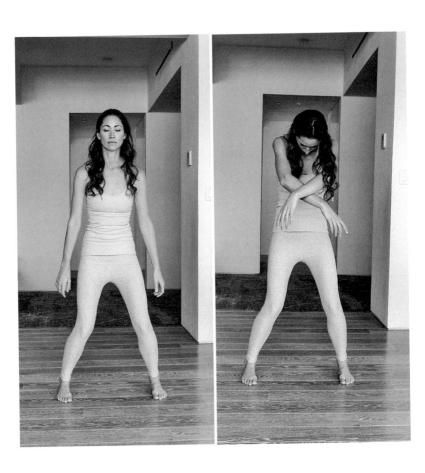

2. Start to shake your arms, really letting them go so you feel your hands and arms wiggle freely. Allow your body to lift and lower naturally in reaction to your breath. Stay with this for 10 long, deep breaths, letting your exhale be a bit longer than your inhale. When you finish, relax your arms by your sides and take a few more long, deep breaths.

3. Cross your arms in front of you and round your back forward a bit like a cat. Relax your head and neck forward. Inhale and bring your body and your arms up through your middle overhead, uncrossing them as you bring them up, so you are

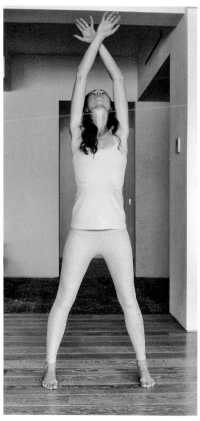 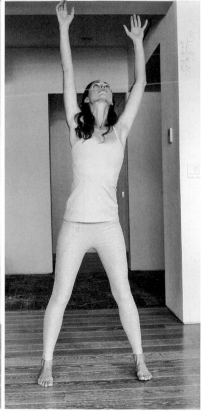

reaching your arms straight upward. Exhale and relax your arms down by your sides. Repeat this 10 times. Come back to your center with your arms relaxed by your sides, and take a few long, deep breaths.

4. Continue standing. In a continuous motion, move your hips and shift your weight onto your right side, keeping your left foot on the ground. Allow your arms to follow along to your right side. Inhale and bring your body and arms out to your right side and up through your center so your arms are straight upward. Exhale and continue the circular motion

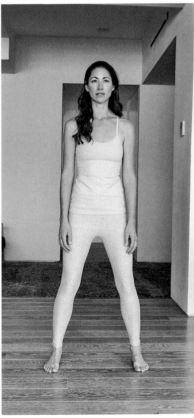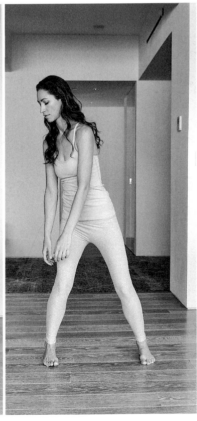

downward and to your left side, bringing your body and arms relaxed over your legs so you are in a forward-bend position. Bend your knees slightly so you are comfortable. Continue the circular motion over to your right side. Inhale and bring your body and arms all the way up so that you are standing upright with your arms overhead. Exhale and come down through center into your forward bend.

5. Continue in this circular motion 4 more times, finishing with your arms straight up. Exhale and relax your arms down by your sides as you stand. Repeat on your left side by moving

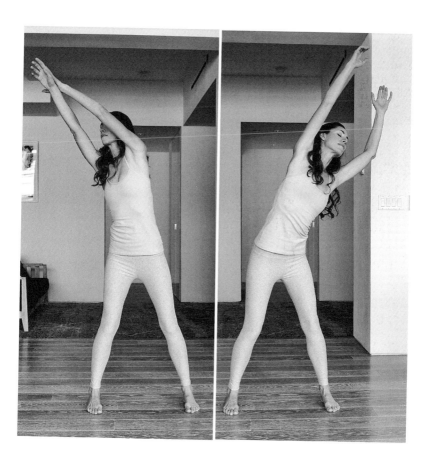

your hips to your left and continuing on in a circular motion. After 4 more repetitions, finish with your arms straight up and then relax them down by your sides. Stay standing for 3 long, deep breaths, and notice how you feel.

6. Maintain your comfortable standing position and take a few long, deep breaths here. Give yourself one more good arm shake and then return to stillness when you finish. Take one long, deep inhale through your nose, then exhale through your mouth.

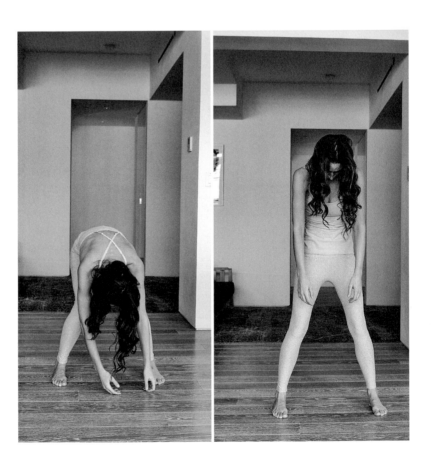

LIFTING GROCERIES

You have just returned from the grocery store or the farmers' market and have set your bag of groceries down on the kitchen floor. Let's take a closer look at the way you would lift that bag of groceries to put them away, and let's see if there are opportunities to move more efficiently that will benefit your body and bring your whole self into harmony. Why are we so interested in the way you lift a bag of groceries? Well, it's because the way you carry out an everyday physical task like this one will likely mirror the tension—or ease—you are bringing to more strenuous activities like running or yoga.

1. Stand next to your bag of groceries. Begin by bending at your knees and bring your hands to the floor for support. Use the strength of your arms, so there is no pressure on your knees at all, and come into a comfortable squat position. Using your arms for support is critical to avoid stress on your knees that can lead to knee problems either suddenly or over time.

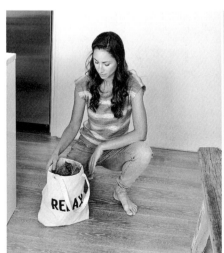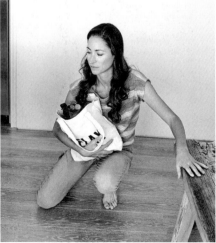

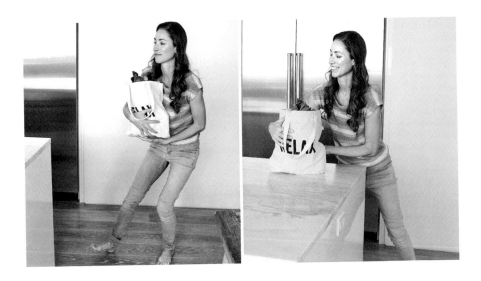

2. Now for lifting the bag: When you open the lid of a jar, do you do it far away from your body, or do you hug it close to you and twist? A close hug usually does the trick. Let's do the same with our groceries. Slide the bag close to you and give it a hug. If it's easy to hug with one arm, support yourself with the other hand on the floor to help yourself up. If the bag is too heavy to lift with one arm, remove one item at a time and place it on the counter until the bag is light enough for you to hug with one arm as you support yourself with the other arm. Place the bag on the counter.

Lifting a bag of groceries in a way that builds whole-body coordination is a practice you can do regularly. This isn't so much about only lifting the bag of groceries in a way that is safe and avoids injury. It's also about moving your whole body in coordination in order to build coordination and strength for other, more challenging physical activities.

SWEEPING THE FLOOR

Sweeping the floor is one of my favorite ways to practice moving well. We might think of cleaning as a dreaded chore or something to outsource while we do more important work. According to tai chi this is a disconnected way of thinking that brings us out of harmony and makes us sick individually and as a society. Also according to tai chi, simple tasks like sweeping and cleaning are part of a practice of simplicity and appreciation of life that brings us vitality.

To sweep in a tai chi, connected way:

1. Bring your broom close to your body. Move yourself from your center as you sweep and use your whole body to move the broom, rather than using just the muscles of your arm and shoulder. The broom moves because your center moves, not because you are pushing it with the force of your arm.

2. Use your arm for guidance of the direction of the broom, not for energy to make the broom move. Pay attention to how you are changing direction, keeping the broom handle close to your body.

If you tend to sweep with one arm, pushing until you feel fatigued in your shoulders or back, you can benefit from this whole-body harmony approach. By bringing more coordination and harmony into your sweeping, it can actually start to feel meditative and pleasurable!

STOP "DOUBLE DOING"

We all have some funky habits and body positions that we fall into, most of which we aren't even aware of. When I get excited about something, I know I tend to hold my arms and hands out and use big, exaggerated gestures. I'm not necessarily going to injure myself with my overly excited hands, but this way of moving builds tension and takes away from whole-self harmony. Tai chi describes alignment as moving in harmony with your whole self every moment along the way. Any action that isn't necessary to complete a movement essentially blocks chi. I don't want to have blocked chi, so I practice relaxing my hands when I'm excited. I feel better and more relaxed, and find it easier to communicate when I'm relaxed as opposed to when I'm doing my tense-handed habit.

I call this extra-hand-motion habit of mine "double doing," because I'm emotionally excited and worked up in my mind, and I "double" that with my body. Many of us do the same thing. When we are excited, we show excitement with our physical gestures. Likewise, when we are frustrated or tense, we double this with our physical gestures. Similarly, double doing can occur when we are exercising—we clench our muscles instead of allowing them to move naturally and efficiently in ways that will benefit our bodies. When I notice that I am double doing, I make a concerted effort to drop my arms, shift into a more relaxed body position, shake things out a bit, and reconnect with my breath. When I come into alignment and harmony, I accomplish more. It's extra motivation to understand that when you "double do," you will experience fatigue more quickly because you're working inefficiently, not because you're building strength so well. It's a useless kind of tired. Dropping the double doing will free up trapped energy and allow your body to gain more strength and a healthier range of motion.

Try this yourself. The next time you are walking along, or hanging out chatting with friends, take note of your body position. Stop whatever you are doing, stand with your feet apart in a wide, grounded stance, soften your knees, and take a few deep breaths.

Notice in this simple standing position how your inhalations lift you, and how your exhalations relax you. Drop your shoulders and your arms, and let your body relax. These adjustments should be so subtle that the people around you don't even notice. Your friends shouldn't even notice that you are doing anything like tai chi or exercising. The secret is moving more efficiently, in a way that will allow you to look and feel more like you, and dissolve bad habits that have been sapping your energy and wearing you out.

Redefining Exercise

I know that you are busy, I totally get it. But "busyness" is not a good reason for failing to make exercise a priority. When exercise is something that we compartmentalize and separate from our other daily tasks, it becomes especially difficult to make the time for it. If you tend to compartmentalize exercise in this way, I want you to shift your thinking. Instead of thinking of exercise as confined to taking a class, going to the gym, or going for a run, redefine exercise as any way that you move your body throughout your whole day. This doesn't mean you should *stop* going to the gym or taking classes or running if these are things that make you feel great. What it means is that you can find ways to move better during overlooked simple moments like walking to work, waiting in line, or cooking. You can also get creative with opportunities to move like taking the stairs instead of the elevator, riding your bike or walking instead of taking a car or train, and creating moments during the day for 5- or 10-minute movement sessions. This applies even if you are a dedicated gym-goer, runner, or yogi. Making it a goal to move more as you go about your daily tasks is always beneficial, whatever your current level of fitness may be.

Life Moments for Movement

Many of us believe that if we manage to get to an exercise class or to the gym after work, we have checked off our "exercise box," and we're good. That gym or class time is beneficial, don't get me wrong, but it's not a substitute for maintaining an active lifestyle beyond the gym, particularly if you work in an office or at a desk job where you are sedentary for most of the day. Modern life can make it tough to get in natural exercise—I get it. But it's important to think beyond designated gym time, to moving our bodies and moving them harmoniously, throughout the entire course of a day. With that in mind, here are some practices to incorporate into your daily routine that extend beyond gym time.

EXERCISES FOR THE OFFICE

Here are some simple exercise routines you can do at the office, or in your home office for a break, if you work from home. All are meant to be done while standing, so you don't have to get down on the floor in your work clothes. Choose the routine that meets your needs, whether you are feeling like a brief strength builder, a stretch for tight hips and back, or an overall mind-body mood boost. I promise that any one of these will do more to boost your mood than an afternoon coffee or sugary snack!

5-Minute Strength and Focus

Here is a simple routine to build strength and focus that you can do right from your office or cubicle. If you are feeling brave, grab some coworkers and do this in a common space!

1. Stand tall with your feet a little wider than hip-width apart. Inhale and lift your body a bit as you bring your hands together in front of you in a prayer position, connected to your body.

2. Exhale and bend your knees, reaching your hips back.

3. Inhale and come back upright. Repeat 20 times.

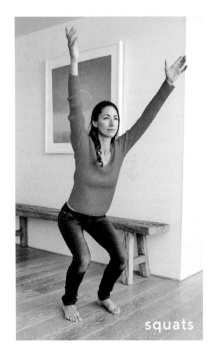

squats

TREE POSE

1. From a standing position, shift your weight onto your right leg and hug your left knee into your chest.

2. Turn your left thigh out so that your lifted knee forms a 90-degree angle, then place the bottom of your left foot on the inside of your right thigh. Alternatively, rest your left toes on the ground with the bottom of your left foot resting against your right inner ankle.

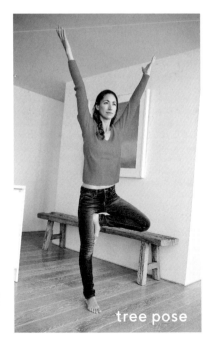

tree pose

3. Reach your arms up over your head in a V-shape. Stay here for 5 long, deep breaths. Repeat on the other side.

Depending on how much time you have, repeat this Squat and Tree Pose series once or twice more.

5-Minute Refresh

Enjoy this feel-good routine to unblock tension in your body and mind. You can do it right at your desk or grab coworkers and do it in a small group.

STANDING SIDE STRETCH

1. Stand tall with your feet slightly apart. Relax your arms by your sides. Take a big inhale and reach your arms up above your head.

2. Exhale and grab hold of your left wrist with your right hand. Inhale and stretch up and slightly over toward your right side.

3. Come back up to center and do the other side. Exhale and relax your arms down by your sides.

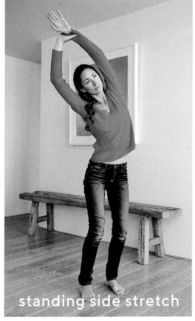

standing side stretch

1. Shift your weight onto your right leg and step your left leg back behind you so that your feet are parallel. Make sure your stance is short and wide enough that you aren't struggling for balance.

2. Inhale and reach your arms up overhead. Exhale and bend your knees while sinking your hips, until your front leg forms a 90-degree angle. You are now in a high lunge.

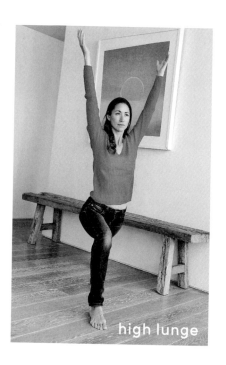

high lunge

3. Inhale and raise your hips as you straighten your legs. Exhale and sink your hips back down. Repeat this movement 3 times. Switch legs and do the same on the other side.

HIGH LUNGE TWIST

1. Come to a high lunge position with your arms up. Exhale and twist toward your right side, opening your arms wide in a T-shape.

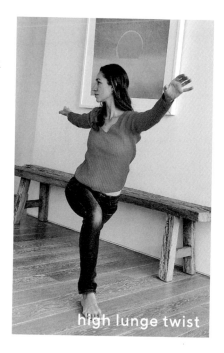

high lunge twist

2. Inhale, straighten up, and come back to a high lunge. Repeat this twisting movement 3 times.

3. Come back to a high lunge. Lean back slightly into your back foot and use the momentum to step your back foot forward to meet your front foot. Relax your arms down by your sides.

4. Repeat on your other side.

Bathroom Break Mood Boost

This mini routine is great when you just need to walk away from your work for a bit to improve how you feel.

COUNTER STRETCH

1. Stand a few feet away from the bathroom counter in a comfortable stance. Bend your knees, round your back slightly, and place your hands on your thighs.

2. Lean to your left and reach for the counter with your right hand, then rest it there. Lean toward your right and reach for

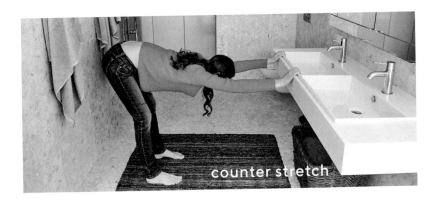

counter stretch

the counter with your left hand, then rest it there. Adjust your stance toward or away from the counter until your arms are straight.

3. Relax your head and neck and stay here for 3 long, deep breaths.

4. To come out of this, look at the counter, walk your feet closer to the counter until you can comfortably stand up tall, and relax your arms by your sides.

SHOULDER STRETCH

1. From a standing position, inhale and reach both arms straight up over your head.

2. Exhale and bend your left arm slightly while clasping your left wrist with your right hand. Lean to your right slightly, shifting your weight to your right foot and pulling gently on your left wrist with your right hand.

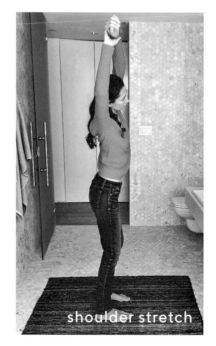

3. Lean farther to your right side and pull on your left wrist until you feel an opening in your left tricep and shoulder.

4. Stay here for 5 long, deep breaths. Relax your arms by your sides and repeat on the other side.

shoulder stretch

EXERCISES WHILE COOKING

Depending on what you are whipping up in the kitchen, there is often downtime while you wait for the oven to preheat or for your smoothie to blend. Use these opportunities to move your body rather than scrolling away on your phone or flipping channels on the TV! Here are a few simple ways to get your blood flowing while you are cooking.

Blender Balancing Act

It's smoothie time, and in the idle moments while you are waiting for your delicious, nutritious concoction to blend, try these moves to give your body (and your appetite) a boost.

TREE POSE

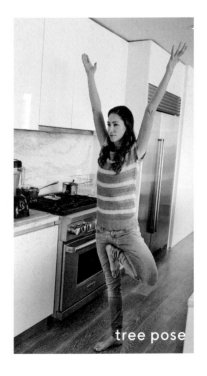

tree pose

1. From a standing position, shift your weight onto your right leg and hug your left knee into your chest.

2. Turn your left thigh out so that your lifted knee forms a 90-degree angle, then place the bottom of your left foot on the inside your right thigh. Alternatively, rest your left toes on the ground with the bottom of your left foot resting against your inner right ankle.

3. Reach your arms up over your head in a V-shape. Stay here for 5 long, deep breaths. Repeat on the other side.

DANCER POSE

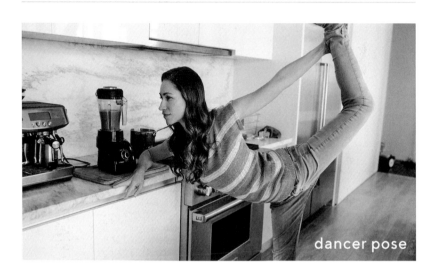

dancer pose

1. Start standing easy. Separate your feet so that they are two fists' distance apart. Shift your weight onto your right leg and hug your left knee into your chest. Drop your left knee toward the ground until you can grab hold of the inside of your left ankle with your left hand.

2. Hang there for a few long, deep breaths to steady your balance. Inhale and press your foot into your hand, creating a bow shape with your bent leg. Lean your opposite arm on the counter for balance.

3. Exhale and relax the bow position a bit. Inhale and press your foot into your hand, tightening your bow. Exhale and relax again. Repeat this process of inhaling and tightening, followed by exhaling and relaxing for a few long, deep breaths. Release

your foot from your hands and squeeze your knee back into your chest and lower your foot to the floor. Repeat on the other side.

PLANK AND CHAIR POSE WAIT AND BAKE

For those longer waits while cooking, here is a pair of strength-building moves that will leave you feeling warmed up and invigorated.

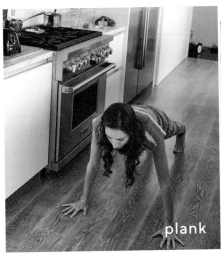
plank

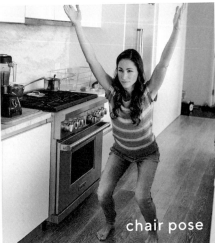
chair pose

1. Come into a plank position. Open your arms a bit wider than you might normally. Shift a bit in your pose from side to side and forward and back.

2. Hang here for 10 long, deep breaths. Inhale and lift your body a bit. Exhale, soften, and move a bit to relax. After 10 breaths, soften your knees to the ground and gently bring yourself up to a standing position.

3. Step with your feet hip-width apart, close your eyes, and reconnect with your breath. Inhale and lift your body and arms

upward. Exhale and sink your hips back into a chair position, leaning forward slightly with your knees bent at 90 degrees, with your back remaining straight.

4. Inhale and return to a comfortable standing position, relaxing your arms down.

5. Repeat 10 times, or for as long as you have until your cooking wait is over! Remember to return to your breath whenever you start to feel tension creeping into your body.

PRIMAL DAILY MOVEMENT

Now that you have shifted your thinking, you should be looking for opportunities to move more wherever you go. Maybe you are in line at the coffee shop or the grocery store or the bank—instead of getting crabby about the long wait, check in with your body and move!

STANDING-IN-LINE BREATH-BODY CONVERSATION

Try this exercise while waiting in line as a way to release both physical and mental tension.

1. Stand with your feet comfortably apart. Soften your knees and your whole body so you aren't rigid. Notice your breath, and the way your inhalations lift you up physically, mentally, and emotionally. Notice the way your exhalations release tension. Breathe deeply and relax your entire body.

2. Move your hips a bit from side to side to relax your back. Move your center toward your left until your left foot steps back slightly. Your body is now open to your left. There is a

difference in moving from your center and leading with your foot. We're practicing moving from the center here.

3. Now move your center forward until your left foot steps forward. Repeat on the other side. (In tai chi, this is a practice of getting out of the way, the idea being that the best way to avoid an attack is to move out of the way of the attacker by moving from your center, rather than moving your arms and legs.)

4. Come back to center and take a few deep breaths, letting your body lift on your inhales and lower on your exhales. Notice what you see around you. This is also a practice of awareness. When you are centered in yourself, you are more aware of what is happening around you.

This practice will make waiting in line more enjoyable and comfortable, and it will improve your mood! I like to think of this practice as not only good for me, but good for everyone around me. The positive vibes ripple outward.

CAR STRETCHES

Of course, focusing on your driving is the most important act when you are behind the wheel, but here are some simple movements you can do safely while sitting in a parked car or stuck in traffic.

SEATED CAT-COW ROLLS

1. Staying seated with your hands on the wheel, exhale and round your lower back into a curve. Then inhale and arch your lower back.

2. Move your ribs toward your right, then curl inward so that your back is rounded, move your ribs toward your left, and then forward into your arch—all in one continuous motion.

3. Repeat this roll 3 times toward the right and 3 times toward the left. Come back to center and take 3 big, deep breaths, letting your body move up slightly as you inhale and down slightly as you exhale.

ZEN TRAVEL MOVES

These simple exercises are great if you travel frequently for work, or for those times when you are on vacation and you're feeling like it's tough to make the time for regular exercise. All can be done easily in a small hotel room.

LUNGE

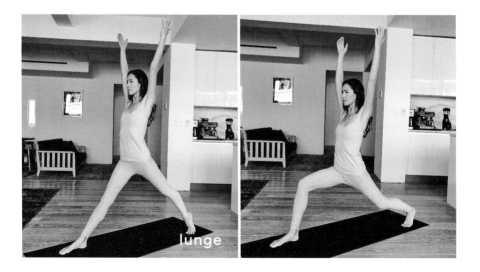

lunge

Lunge:

1. Start standing. Shift your hips from side to side to find a comfortable position.

2. Shift your weight to your right side and slide your left leg behind you into a lunge position. Keep your feet wide enough apart to maintain a steady balance and your arms relaxed by your sides. Exhale and sink your hips toward the floor while softening both knees into a lunge.

3. Inhale and gently straighten both knees to lift your hips while raising your arms up toward the ceiling.

4. Exhale and sink back into your lunge. Repeat 10 times with your breath. Switch sides and repeat with the opposite leg in front.

Lunge with knee lift:

1. Begin your second set of lunges, but this time when you inhale and come up, pick up your back foot and hug your knee into your chest with a squeeze.

2. Exhale as you lower your raised leg back into your lunge.

3. Repeat 10 times with your breath. Switch legs and repeat with the opposite leg in front.

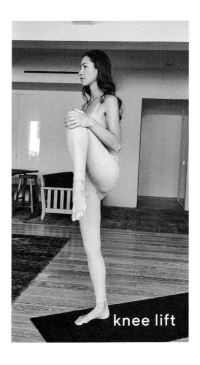

knee lift

1. Sit on the ground with your legs stretched out in front of you. Bend your knees to create a diamond shape with your legs, bringing the bottoms of your feet together, knees out to your sides. Lean back until your hands catch you on the ground behind you.

2. Inhale and let your chest lift and fill with your breath. Exhale and curl your back, bringing your torso forward over your legs. Hang here for 10 long, deep breaths, shifting your body as needed into any spaces that feel tight or stuck.

3. Roll yourself back up. Lean into your right hip and slide your left leg straight behind you. Your right leg remains bent in front of you, so that you come into a relaxed pigeon position. Inhale and lean back a bit. Exhale and relax your body forward over your front leg. Hang here for 10 long, deep breaths, shifting as necessary into any spaces in your body that feel tight or stuck.

4. Roll back up, lean into your right hip, and slide your left leg around, bringing your feet together again. Repeat on your other side. Do this 5 times on each side.

Exercise Routines: ENERGIZE and RESTORE

On the following pages, I've outlined some wellness routines for you to pick and choose from, depending on what your body needs and how you want to feel on any given day. Go for ENERGIZE if you are feeling sluggish and want a pick-me-up, or if you are feeling like you have excess energy that you need to burn off. Go for RESTORE when you are feeling tired or burned out and want to unplug and take things down a notch. These routines involve a mix of exercise, yoga, walking, breathing, and meditation, and they can be done at any time of day.

ENERGIZE

Energizing Yoga Flow

This routine includes several yoga poses put together in sequence to form a short flow that you can repeat several times to build energy. It finishes off with some centering breathing exercises.

WARRIOR 2—HOLD

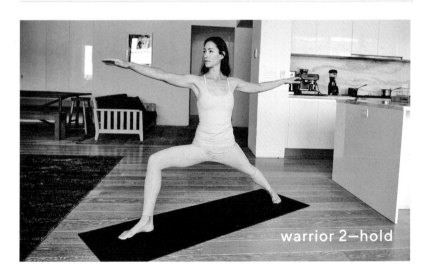

1. Stand with your feet wide apart in a straddle position. Turn your right toes forward and turn your left toes in slightly.

Inhale and lift your arms up and out to the sides to form a T-shape.

2. Exhale and sink your hips low, bending your front knee over your front ankle at a 90-degree angle. Keep your back knee a bit soft.

3. Hang here for 10 long, deep breaths. Let each inhale lift you up, and let each exhale sink you a bit farther down into the position.

WARRIOR 2—LIFT AND LOWER

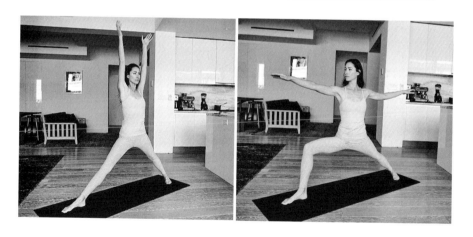

1. Inhale and straighten your legs while raising your arms above your head. Exhale and sink back down into Warrior 2, with your front knee bent and your arms lowering back into a T-shape.

2. Repeat this 3 times, moving with your breath.

3. Switch sides and repeat, starting with Warrior 2—Hold.

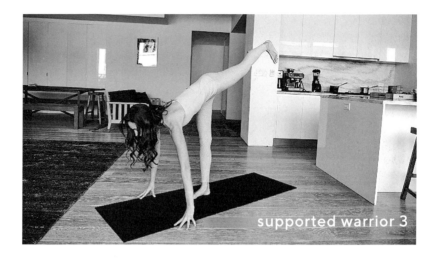

1. Stand with your feet hip-width apart. Bend your knees slightly and bring your body forward over your front right standing leg.

2. Lift your left leg off the ground, so your standing right leg and lifted left leg form a 90-degree angle.

3. Bring your fingertips to the ground in front of you for balance. Hang here for 5 long, deep breaths. Repeat on the other side.

SUPPORTED WARRIOR 3—ROLL-UP

1. From Supported Warrior 3, bend your knees and round your back. Inhale and lift your torso so that you are standing on your right leg while hugging your left knee into your chest.

2. Exhale and send your left leg behind you while leaning your torso forward into Warrior 3, allowing your hands to touch the ground again for support.

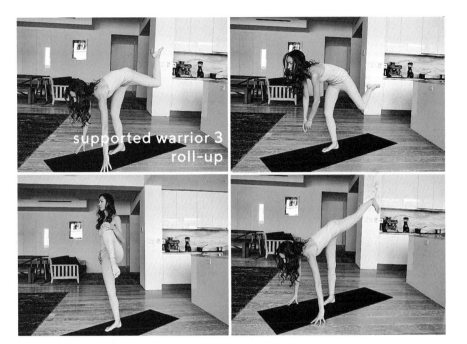

supported warrior 3
roll-up

3. Inhale and lift your torso again while hugging your left knee to your chest. Repeat 10 times with your breath. Switch sides and repeat, starting with Supported Warrior 3.

PLANK INTO CHILD'S POSE

1. From a standing position, bring your hands to the ground in front of you, bend your knees, and step back into a plank position. Shift a bit from side to side and from front to back to relax your body and to let some of the effort go. Hang here for 10 long, deep breaths.

2. Lower your knees to the ground and relax your hips to your heels into Child's Pose. Rest your arms by your sides. Stay here for 5 long, deep breaths. Repeat 5 times.

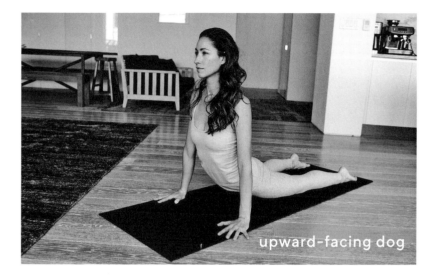

upward-facing dog

1. Beginning in plank pose, bend your elbows and lower your entire body slowly toward the ground. Straighten your arms behind you.

2. Once you are lying fully on the ground, rock your hips a bit from side to side. Bend your elbows again with your palms flat against the ground to the sides of your chest.

3. With your palms, push your torso upward, straightening your elbows while keeping your hips on the ground, until you reach a place where you feel a good opening in your back but no pain.

4. Taking several long, deep breaths, allow your head, neck, and shoulders to relax. Repeat 5 times.

1. Sit in a comfortable position, either on the ground or in a chair. Close your eyes and bring your attention to your breath.

2. Let your body lift up with each inhale. Let your body soften and relax with each exhale. Stay here for 20 long, deep breaths.

walking chi wake-up

During the day to keep your energy up and your blood flowing, walk as much as possible. Take a break and go outside for a brisk walk for at least 20 minutes at a time. If you like to alternate jogging and walking, that's great, too. Try to do this first thing in the morning, for a break in the afternoon around lunch, and sometime in the evening—perhaps right after work.

RESTORE

Restorative Yoga Flow

This routine includes a number of moves put together into a short flow that you can repeat several times to relax your body and restore when you are feeling depleted or tired. It closes with a calming breathing exercise.

1. Sit however is most comfortable for you. Close your eyes and notice your breathing. Let your inhale lift your body a bit. Allow your exhale to lower and relax you a bit.

2. Shift your body gently and make adjustments as necessary to be more comfortable. Notice any places that feel a bit stuck or tense. Move your body toward these areas, whether that means leaning forward to release tension in your lower back or walking your hands behind you to open up your shoulders and chest. Take a few deep breaths here and notice any changes.

3. Bring yourself gently back to center. Stay here for 5 minutes, or 5 sets of 10 long, deep breaths.

ONE LEG OUT SIDE STRETCH

1. From a seated cross-legged position, lean to your left side and extend your right leg out to your right side.

2. Lean toward your right leg in a side stretch and relax your right forearm on the ground in front of your right leg for support. Shift your body around in this position, focusing on any spaces that feel tight or tense.

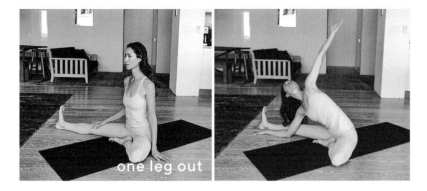

one leg out

3. Reach your left arm up and overhead toward your right foot, if that feels like a nice stretch for you. Stay here for 5 long, deep breaths. Bring yourself upright again and repeat on the other side.

BOTH LEGS OUT SIDE STRETCH

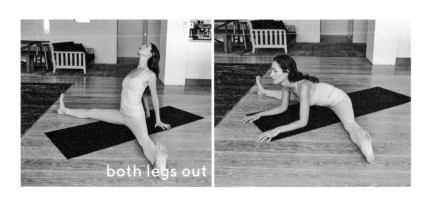

both legs out

1. Bring both legs out to your sides in a comfortable straddle position. Lean back and place your hands on the ground behind you for support.

2. Inhale, filling your lungs with breath and opening your torso toward the ceiling. Exhale and round your back, crawling

your torso forward toward the floor, placing your forearms on the ground in front of you.

3. On your forearms, walk your torso over to your right and then to your left, searching for places that are tight and that need attention. Stay with this for 10 long, deep breaths, and then gently bring yourself back upright.

BOTH LEGS FORWARD RELAX

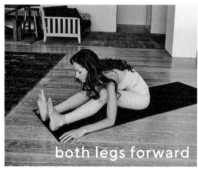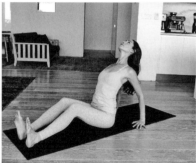

both legs forward

1. Stretch both legs out in front of you, keeping a slight bend in your knees. Lean back and bring your hands to the ground behind you for support.

2. Inhale and raise your torso upward. Exhale and lean forward, relaxing your torso, head, and neck over your legs. Let your body move gently from side to side to find places that are tight and that could use your attention.

3. Stay with this for 10 long, deep breaths. Gently bring your torso upright. Repeat 5 times.

1. Roll down to rest on your back. Take a few long, deep breaths here and check in with your body. Hug your knees into your chest. Rock gently a bit from side to side on your back.

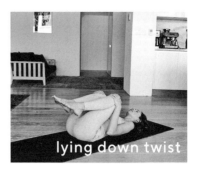

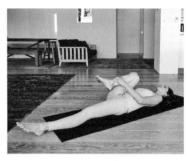

lying down twist

2. Drop your knees to the right side until they rest on the ground. Open your arms out to your sides in a T-shape and either look up at the ceiling or over your left shoulder, if that feels like a good stretch.

3. Stay with this for 10 long, deep breaths. Repeat on the other side. Do this 5 times for each side.

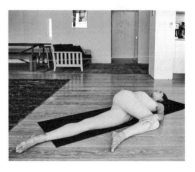

LYING DOWN BREATHING EXERCISE TO CLOSE

1. Lie down flat on your back and relax your arms out to your sides. Take a few long, deep breaths in through your nose and out through your mouth.

2. Rest here for 5 minutes or 5 sets of 10 long, deep breaths. When you are ready, gently bring yourself back up to sitting.

walking meditation to restore

Get outside for a slow, reflective walk. Try not to have a plan or a destination. Leave your phone at home and let your mind focus on your breath. Take breaks as needed to stand still or to sit on the ground and just be with yourself and reflect. Try to do this, for at least 20 minutes at a time, first thing in the morning, at some point midday, and in the evening.

Getting Outside

The art of healing comes from nature, not from the physician.
—Paracelsus

At one time or another, we've all experienced the healing power of getting outside for a walk in the woods or on the beach, or simply watching the sunset. But in the hustle and bustle of our daily lives, we forget that this key to feeling better, more connected, and less stressed is just outside our front door. Research shows that exposure to green space reduces the risk of life-threatening health issues including cardiovascular disease, type 2 diabetes, and high blood pressure. As a culture we are finally catching on with trends like forest bathing, doctors writing prescriptions for time spent in parks and in nature, and more urban green spaces. Beyond putting our phones down to manage screen time, we need to head outdoors to genuinely replenish.

SEASONAL MOVEMENT

Just as the weather and the natural world around us changes with each season, so should the way we exercise and move our bodies. In winter, let yourself wind down, rest, restore, and appreciate all that the past year has brought to your life. In spring, allow yourself to be reborn, reinvent yourself, come out of your shell, and explore. In summer, allow yourself to melt and be mellow, enjoy being outside, savor the energy of long days, play until you need to rest, then play again. In fall, allow yourself to regain focus with the crispness of the air, and create a fresh, new, productive routine that supports your goals.

Take a moment to reflect on the current season. What are your personal goals and how can you allow the season to support you? What does the air feel like outside where you are, and how does the weather of this season affect you? What is the general mood or energy you sense from nature and people during this time? How can you bring yourself more in tune with the particular season you're in?

Winter Wonder Walks

Most of us tend to stay inside during the winter, jetting from one indoor place to the next to avoid the cold. But we can use the cold to invigorate us and form a completely different relationship with winter by bundling up for a pleasure walk.

1. Dress warmly in layers and bring a small blanket or towel (that you don't mind getting a bit dirty) along with you. Focus on

your breathing as you walk and notice how the cold air feels moving in and out of you.

2. Walk to an outdoor spot where you can sit comfortably for a few minutes, maybe a bench or somewhere on the ground. Sit on the blanket you brought if you are opting for the ground.

3. Sit down, close your eyes, and notice how you feel. Allow the cold air to invigorate you. Welcome it in as nourishment, instead of something to avoid. Stay here for 10 long, deep breaths. Move around gently in some side-to-side stretches and allow your body to be invigorated by the air.

4. When you're ready, gently come to a comfortable standing position. Relax your arms by your sides and shake your arms in a Tai Chi Wake and Shake (see page 184) to wake up your chi. Continue to shake your arms for 5 long, deep breaths and then rest in a calm, steady stance. Notice how you feel. Head back inside when you are ready.

Spring Rebirth Routine

Here is a simple springtime routine to get your energy levels up and your blood moving. Head out into nature to do this routine, whether that's out in your yard or to a local park. The following exercises should be done in succession on one side, then repeated on the other side.

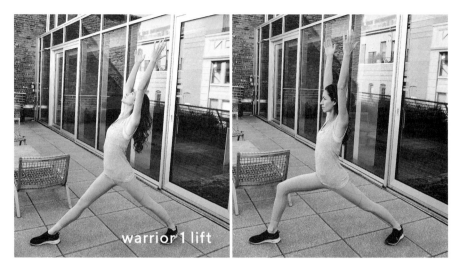

warrior 1 lift

1. Stand with your feet hip-width apart. Shift your weight onto your right leg and step your left leg back.

2. With your right toes pointing forward, angle your left toes out 45 degrees while keeping your hips square.

3. Inhale and raise your arms up overhead while lifting your hips up so that your legs straighten.

4. Exhale and sink your hips, bending your front knee. Repeat 4 more times on this side.

LOW LUNGE TWIST

1. From a standing position, bring your hands to the ground, bending your knees slightly. Lean to your right and bring your

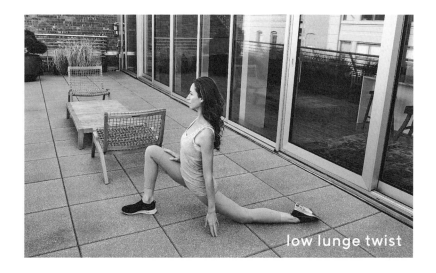

low lunge twist

left leg back to a low lunge. Gently lower your left knee to the ground.

2. Inhale and bring your torso upright and arch back slightly.

3. Exhale and twist toward your front leg, bringing your left hand to your right knee and your right hand to your back leg.

4. Bring your body back toward your low lunge and gently change sides. Repeat twice on each side.

WARRIOR 3 ROLL-UPS

1. From a standing position, bring your hands to the ground in front of you, lift your hips a bit, and shift your weight to your front right leg so that your left leg comes off the ground parallel with the floor. Keep your hands on the ground in front of you for support.

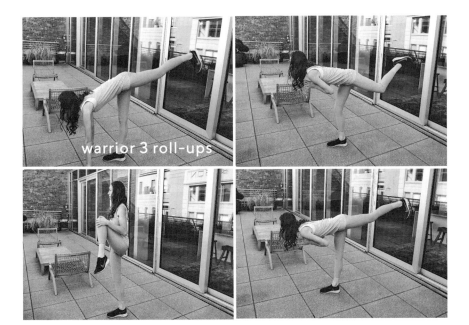

warrior 3 roll-ups

2. Bend both knees, inhale, and roll up to standing, hugging your left knee into your chest. Exhale and come back down, bringing your hands to the ground in front of you and your left leg behind you, parallel to the ground.

3. Repeat this roll-up, up and down, 9 more times on this side.

Come back to a standing position and repeat the entire Spring Rebirth Routine on the other side, beginning with Warrior 1 Lifts.

Summer Soak-Up Practice

This is a great, cooling routine that is perfect for warm summer temps. It will relax your entire body and help to open up and release your back.

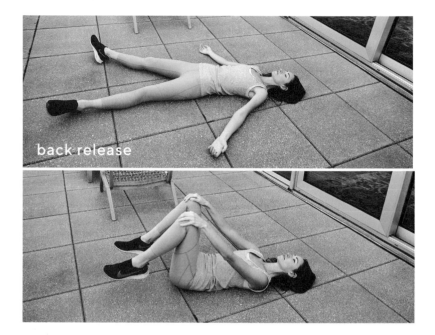

back release

1. Lie flat on your back on a comfortable surface. Hug your knees into your chest and bring your hands to the tops of your knees. Let the weight of your legs relax away from you.

2. This should feel like a nice stretch from the top of your head down through your tailbone. Take 3 long, deep breaths here.

EASY TWIST

1. Lie on your back and hug both knees into your chest. Rock a bit from side to side to release your back.

2. Relax both knees over toward your right side until your right knee touches the ground. Open your arms out to your sides in a T-shape. Take 10 long, deep breaths here.

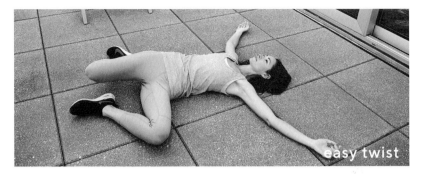

easy twist

3. Bring your knees back to center and then do the same on your left side. Return to center.

BRIDGE

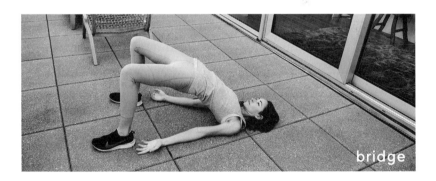

bridge

1. Lie on your back with your knees bent comfortably and with your arms straight along the ground beside you, so that your fingertips just touch your heels.

2. Press your feet into the ground and lift your hips up above you, creating an arch in your back. Hang here for 5 long, deep breaths and then slowly roll down.

3. Rest for 3 long, deep breaths, then repeat twice more.

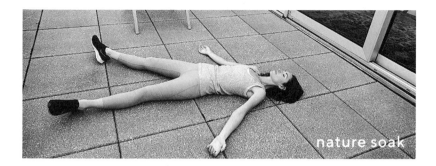

1. Lie on your back and relax with your legs stretched out in front of you and your arms by your sides, or with your hands on your belly if that's more comfortable for you.

2. Rest here for 3 minutes or so, observing the nature around you. Notice how the air feels, any sounds you hear, and anything you see. Watch the clouds go by and take note of how you feel.

Flying Fall Flow

This is a great routine for harnessing the crisp energy of fall. Use this routine to refocus and align with your goals.

STANDING SWINGS

1. Stand with your feet hip-width apart, arms by your sides. Bend your knees slightly. Inhale and swing your arms forward and up above your head.

2. Exhale and swing your arms downward and slightly back, while keeping your knees soft.

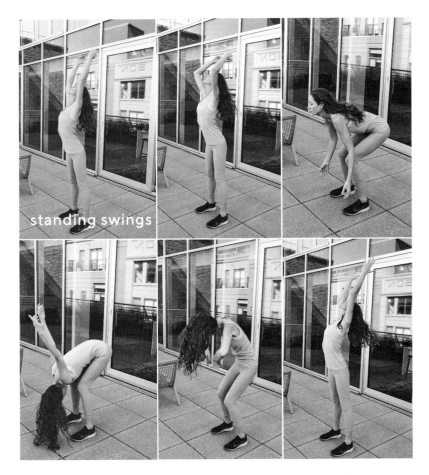

standing swings

3. Repeat this swinging motion 10 times. On your tenth repetition, hold your breath in with your arms up for a slow count of 5. Exhale and relax your arms down. Come back to your center stance and take a few long, deep breaths.

RAINBOW STRETCH

1. Start standing. Bend your knees slightly. Take a big inhale and stretch your arms overhead.

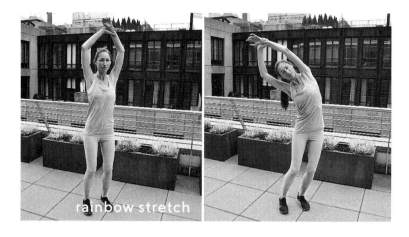
rainbow stretch

2. Grab your right wrist with your left hand as you exhale. Inhale and stretch up and over toward your left like a rainbow. Hang here for a few long, deep breaths.

3. Come back to center and then do the same on your other side.

HOEDOWN KNEE LIFTS

1. Start standing. Shift your weight onto your left leg. Take a big inhale and hug your right knee into your chest.

2. Exhale and place your foot back down, then shift your weight onto your right leg. Inhale and hug your left knee into your chest. Exhale and place your foot down.

3. Continue this movement, 10 times on each side. If you want an extra burst of energy, turn it into a hop switch instead of a standing switch with your legs.

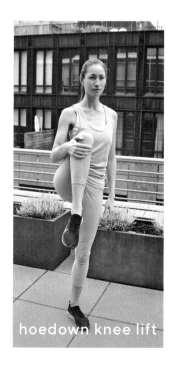
hoedown knee lift

journal it out:
feel-good body goals

It's time to revisit the questions you asked yourself at the start of Week 4 and take stock of the progress you've made. Jot down your responses as you reflect on the questions and compare your answers to those you recorded previously.

- How many times this week did you engage in structured exercise, like practicing yoga, going for a hike, or taking an exercise class? Going forward, how many times a week would you ideally like to be able to exercise?

- During exercise this week, what was happening in your mind? Were you carrying mental stress and negativity with you into your workouts?

- What new kinds of exercise did you do this week? Which of these would you be open to incorporating into your routine long-term?

- Over the past week, did you tend to stay moving throughout the course of each day, or did you spend more time being sedentary?

- Did you find new opportunities to move more over the course of this week? Did you take the stairs instead of the elevator? Get up from your desk at work more often to take walks? Squeeze in a few planks or stretching during your downtime? If so, how did this make you feel?

Based on your new answers to these questions, what are some changes that you would like to make to the way you approach exercise and moving your body?

People Who Are Living It Right

MIKE TAYLOR
*Cofounder of Strala Yoga, on Moving Well as a
Strategy for Life*

I met my husband and business partner, Mike, at a yoga retreat, and
what drew me to him was how he moved. It wasn't just that he could
do all kinds of crazy-difficult yoga moves; it was that he could do
them with such ease—nothing was forced. Mike and I come from
two very different worlds. I'm a farm girl and he was top of his class
at Exeter, Harvard, and Oxford. He studied mind-body medicine
at Harvard and complementary medicine at Oxford. His area of expertise is East Asian martial and healing arts. But we have yoga in
common, and we practice for a lot of the same reasons: connection,
community, and well-being. We also see a lot of the same problems
with yoga: dogma, abuse, and rigidity. We ended up creating a business and a whole world together based on our common approach
and shared vision when it comes to these issues.

When we first met, you ran a start-up and practiced
yoga as a hobby. How has your approach to self-care and
movement changed since then? What do you recommend
for people who spend a lot of time in an office and want to
move well?

When I was younger, practices like yoga were a hobby for me,
separate from other parts of my life. Now they're the main course.
Not because I'm doing yoga or tai chi all the time; life is mostly
too busy for that. But now I focus less on the forms, more on the
foundations. I don't have to be doing a yoga pose to be doing yoga

or wait for yoga-time to feel better. I always try to be practicing in some way, through how I sit or stand, walk, run, climb stairs, or connect with people in a meeting.

This is helpful to keep in mind if you spend many hours of the day in an office, or a car, or at home with your kids. Wherever you are, you can always practice three things: movability, connection, and harmony.

How do you find time for movement during the day while juggling the workload of managing Strala, teaching, traveling, and being a dad?

We're all busy. And it's wonderful if we can find an hour, or even just 5 minutes, just to practice in a special way, in some special place. But even more important, I think it's best when what we practice isn't limited to special times and places. It's very difficult to undo in a few minutes what we do with ourselves all day long. So what we do all day long is what matters most.

Every night, I carry Daisy to bed and we walk around the room a bit first, singing a few songs. And on many days, this is where I'm practicing tai chi the most, moving my whole body from my belly, pulling weight out of one leg, then the other, walking forward, back, side to side, making circles. All of it is exactly how I'd get around if I was moving with another person in tai chi.

And throughout the day, there are always a few moments to drop down for some whole-body lift-ups, which are much more fun than push-ups. The start of this practice is by lifting first from your center rather than just pushing the floor away with your shoulders and arms, and also rolling this movement from side to side, so it's not just a straight, linear up and down.

You can find opportunities to move your body in whatever

form your life takes. That's something that's very special, and very valuable. It makes all of your time your own.

What's one simple practice we can do every day to move better and feel better?

Breathe. But not as something separate from the rest of you. Breathe deeply in connection with your whole body, so that your breath moves you. And move, but not as a collection of parts separate from each other, and separately controlled. Move as one whole you, guided almost entirely, let's say the first 90 percent, from your center.

TRAINER JOE DOWDELL
on Eating Well, Sleeping Well, and Doing the Workouts You Enjoy

Joe Dowdell is a professional trainer who owns his own gym, Peak Performance, in NYC. He gave me my first gig teaching yoga in his gym to his training staff. I have always been incredibly grateful to him for that first opportunity, and for his friendship and guidance over the years. I'm honored to share some of his insights with you here.

What is the most important thing we can do to stay physically strong and balanced?

First and foremost, the most important thing you can do is to get a good night's sleep (i.e., 6 to 8 hours). Sleep sets the stage for performance, whether it's at work, in the gym, at the yoga studio, or just in your daily activities, by allowing your body and brain to function properly. In addition, sleep can affect your hormones, including the hormones that control appetite regulation, ghrelin and leptin. Ghrelin increases appetite and leptin decreases it. With a lack of sleep, ghrelin production increases and leptin decreases, which can be a recipe for bad nutritional choices.

Which leads me to the next most important thing you can do, and that is to properly fuel your body with nutrient-dense foods, especially lean sources of protein, fibrous vegetables and fruits, and some good fat. And drink plenty of water (½ to 1 ounce of water per pound of body weight per day, depending on your activity level).

Finally, you should try to do some sort of physical activity every day, whether it's a structured workout that is moderate to high intensity, a morning or evening walk, or even something nontraditional like gardening.

What is your personal routine for staying well?

During the week, I start my day either at five or six A.M., depending on my personal training schedule. First thing for me is some coffee, before I hit my computer to answer emails and then catch up on the news. Then I feed and walk my dog and have some breakfast before heading out to the studio to train my morning clients. After I'm done with my morning clients, I will usually do my personal workout, which, depending on the day, will either be a strength-training session or a boxing/kickboxing session. I typically train myself six days a week, and sometimes if I'm feeling really good, I may get in a second workout (i.e., extra cardio) on the same day.

At lunchtime, I head home to feed and walk my dog, have some lunch, and do some computer work before heading back to the gym to train a couple of afternoon clients. Once I'm done with my clients for the day, I'll head back home, spend some time working on other projects, and then either cook some dinner or go out for a bite to eat with friends. Finally, I will usually relax for a couple of hours by watching some sports or a movie before walking my dog one last time, and I'm usually in bed by ten thirty P.M.

Should we vary our workouts with the seasons, and how?

The change of seasons can offer unique opportunities to add things into your routine, such as running outside, hiking, surfing, skiing, etc. Being able to get outside is always a bonus when it comes to being active, as sunshine, fresh air, and even a change of scenery can be potent positive stimuli for the brain and the body.

How do we know what workouts are best for us, and how do we put together a workout schedule that is most beneficial?

Ultimately, I think the best workout is always going to be the one that a person enjoys and is willing to do consistently. Honestly, the same thing applies to nutrition as well. I can give someone a really well-thought-out workout plan and have my nutritionist give them an amazing nutritional plan, but if the person isn't willing to commit to it because they either don't enjoy it or find it too difficult to follow, they're not going to get the results they are looking for. Consistency is really important for long-term success, and from my experience, if someone doesn't like a particular workout or nutritional plan, they're eventually going to quit. On the other hand, if they really enjoy it or find it convenient to implement into their life, they will be much more consistent.

clean
living
for life

living well

rue well-being is much simpler than we make it out to be. Notice that I did not say that it's easy, but simple. Well-being is about cultivating the daily practices and embracing the ancient wisdom that are already inside of you! Instead of taking something to help you sleep, let's address the reasons you aren't sleeping well. Instead of collecting drawers full of yoga pants, let's find the yoga inside ourselves. Instead of eating junk food or scrolling mindlessly when we are bored, let's reach out to others and reconnect with ourselves. The key is learning to subtract, rather than to add. We must slow down in order to pay attention to our thoughts and our true intentions and to listen to our bodies and our minds. Layering on green juices and fitness classes without searching within won't cut it.

Once, as I was walking down the street in New York City, a woman caught my attention. She was dressed in sweaty gym clothes, carrying a tote bag from the branded fitness class she had just attended, and gulping down a smoothie while perched over a garbage can. She proceeded to toss out the drink's packaging within fifteen seconds or so, before rushing off to wherever it was she was headed next. I'm not making an example of this woman to be cruel—we have all been there! We are all guilty of this kind of behavior, in one way or another. We think that wellness is about pushing ourselves harder and constantly doing more. I am here to challenge that notion. I believe that un-busying ourselves might be the most challenging and the most effective rebellious wellness act. We need to use our self-discipline to simplify our lives.

Now that you have come to the end of your 28-day *Clean Mind, Clean Body* detox, take a moment to congratulate yourself. The very act of embarking on this challenge, and sticking with it for 28 days, even if you deviated from the plan occasionally, is a huge accomplishment. You committed to change, and you may not realize it, but you are already living a life that is the reflection of your new habits. The secret is the simplicity of these activities, allowing them to find their way into your day, and, most important, adjusting and tailoring them to feel like you. This isn't about punishment, restricting, or overexercising yourself to see results. It's about slowing down, simplifying, and allowing the real you to emerge through these practices. That's clean living for life.

Daily Wellness Routines

Your initial detox period is over, and hopefully you feel fantastic. Now we want to keep that feeling going! Let's find a way to do that together with some sample Daily Wellness Routines that you can begin to follow just as soon as your 28-day detox is over. These routines are just examples of what you might do. Feel free to modify them to meet your needs and suit your schedule, or to create your own unique combinations from the practices outlined in this book.

I've divided these sample routines into "Weekdays" and "Weekends," because most of us have very different flows to these days. Weekdays, as I designate them, are your busier and less flexible days, even if those days are not Monday through Friday for you— they are not always for me. Weekends, as I designate them, are your days with more free time and downtime, even if those days are not Saturday and Sunday in your schedule. I also give you options for ENERGIZING versus RESTORATIVE Weekdays and Weekends, which you can choose from depending on your energy levels, whether you are feeling fantastic or fighting a cold, and whether you need a bit of a boost or want to mellow out. If your life looks different than the usual 5-day week, 2-day weekend schedule, adjust my recommendations as necessary to meet your needs. And most important, listen to what your body is telling you.

WEEKDAYS

ENERGIZING Weekday Routine

Morning

Upon Waking: Morning Tai Chi Wake and Shake (see page 184)

Clean Mind Practice: Make Your Bed (see page 26)

Clean Mind Practice: Setting an Intention for Your Day (see page 88)

Clean Body Recipe: Extra Oat-y Ginger Cinnamon Oatmeal (see page 144)

Afternoon

Clean Mind Practice: Invite Colleagues to Lunch!—Eating with community is better for your well-being than eating alone. You'll expand your comfort zone and probably get inspired by getting to know your colleagues a bit more.

Clean Mind Practice: Office Space Cleanse—Take a bit of time to clean the clutter from your office space.

Evening

Clean Body Recipe: Magic Masala Rice and Veggies (see page 154)—Cook with friends or family.

Clean Mind Practice: Reflective Journaling (see page 54)

Bedtime Routine: Deep Belly Breathing (see page 33)

RESTORATIVE Weekday Routine

Morning

Upon Waking: Meditation for Work-Life Harmony (see page 38)

Clean Mind Practice: Make Your Bed (see page 26)

Clean Body Recipe: Turmeric Latte (see page 136) or Iced Mint Sun Tea (see page 139), depending on the season

Afternoon

Clean Mind Practice: Afternoon Walk and Reflection Time (see page 40)

Clean Body Practice: Bathroom Break Mood Boost (see page 198)

Evening

Clean Mind Practice: Restorative Yoga Flow (see page 213)

Bedtime Routine: Deep Belly Breathing (see page 33)

WEEKENDS

ENERGIZING Weekend Routine

Morning

Upon Waking: Meditation for a Healing Space (see page 24)

Clean Body Practice: Energizing Yoga Flow (see page 208)

Clean Mind Practice: Make Your Bed (see page 26)

Clean Mind Practice: Closet Cleanse (see page 25)

Afternoon

Clean Body Recipe: Calm the Vata Veggie Soup (page 148)

Clean Mind Practice: Pantry Deep Clean (see page 27)

Clean Body Practice: Eat with the Season (see page 131)

Clean Body Practice: Lifting Groceries (see page 189)

Evening

Clean Mind Practice: Reflective Journaling (see page 54)

Bedtime Routine: "Be Moved" Meditation Practice (see page 55)

RESTORATIVE Weekend Routine

Morning

Upon Waking: Morning Yoga and Meditation (see page 37)

Clean Mind Practice: Make Your Bed (see page 26)

Clean Mind Practice: Cleaning with Kids (see page 21)

Afternoon

Clean Mind Practice: Alone Time (see page 53)

Clean Mind Practice: Reflective Journaling (see page 54)

Evening

Clean Body Recipe: Calm the Vata Veggie Soup (see page 148)

Clean Mind Practice: DIY Bathroom Spa and Pleasure Reading (see pages 85 and 86)

Bedtime Routine: "Be Moved" Meditation Practice (see page 55)

THANK YOU FOR TAKING this journey with me. I hope these new healthy habits have already made a home in you and that they will inspire a cascade of good in your life. The goal isn't perfection or becoming an expert in ancient wisdom. The goal is to remain an absolute beginner, to constantly fine-tune and adapt, and to use these ancient practices made new to live your best life. The power of this ancient wisdom is already inside you, just waiting to be activated. You have to practice, every day. It's not easy, but it's simple. Stay on the path. When you stray, come back to just one practice, every day, until you find your rhythm again.

acknowledgments

Thank you, Linda Loewenthal, for your mentorship, patient encouragement, and representation. Jessica Sindler, thank you for the opportunity, your vision, and trust. For my contributors, Courtney Nichols Gould, Shelah Bergbower, Mallika Chopra, Rabbi Jonathan Blake, Jasmine Hemsley, Dr. Robin Berzin, Joe Dowdell, and Mike Taylor, thank you for sharing your wisdom that we all can learn from in the book, and for your support on my personal journey. Thank you to the entire team at Dey Street, including Kendra Newton, Anna Brill, Alivia Lopez, and Sharyn Rosenblum.

Sam Berlind, thank you for being a human encyclopedia of the East Asian Arts and making me feel like I can do anything. Thank you Mike (you get two lines here) for having long breakfasts and bike rides and snuggle time with Daisy so I can write, reflect, and try to do some good with this work. Thank you also for teaching me some of those ninja skills, even though you don't like when I call them that. *Clean Mind Clean Body*, like all projects, is a group effort, and I'm honored to be a member of this team.

index

Ginger (*cont.*)
  health benefits, 128
  Turmeric Banana Mango Nice
    Cream, 143
  Turmeric Banana Mango
    Smoothie, 142
  Turmeric Latte, 136
  Turmeric Smashed Potatoes,
    153
Glass Cleaner, 24
Goals
  establishing, 13–16
  feel-good, journaling, 14,
    178–79
  feel-good body goals, 229
  for life, revisiting, 43
  spiritual, 71–73
Gould, Courtney Nichols, 58–61
Groceries, lifting, 189–90
Grocery shopping, 129

H

Habits
  changing, 13, 181
  food-related, 103–5
  healthy, 68
Health issues, 167–68
Hemsley, Jasmine, 162–66
Herbs. *See also specific herbs*
  Ayurvedic, 109
High lunge, 197
High lunge twist, 197–98

Hip release, 207
Hobbies, cultivating, 41
Hoedown knee lifts, 228
Homemade Coconut Whipped
  Cream, 138
House cleanse, 22–24
"How Can I Serve?" meditation,
  80–81

I

Iced Mint Sun Tea, 139
Inflammation, 75
Inner self, staying connected
  with, 52–54
Inspiration walks, 53–54
Insula, 75–76
Insulin, 126
Intent.com, 91–92
Intention, living with, 87–91
Intention-setting, 90–91, 93–94
Intermittent fasting, 126–27

J

Journaling, 5
  eating habits, 104–5
  feel-good body goals, 178–79,
    229
  feel-good goals, 14
  reflective, 54
  spiritual goal setting, 73

about the author

TARA STILES is a wellness expert, bestselling author, and the founder of Strala Yoga. The Strala approach combines yoga, tai chi, and traditional Chinese and Japanese medicine to help people release stress, heal, let go of negative habits, and move more easily through everyday challenges. Tara's bestselling books, which have been translated and published in multiple languages, include *Strala Yoga*, *Make Your Own Rules Diet*, *Yoga Cures*, and *Slim Calm Sexy Yoga*, and she has been featured in the *New York Times*, *Vogue*, *Elle*, *Harper's Bazaar*, *InStyle*, *Esquire*, and *Shape*. Tara's work has been used in a case study by Harvard University; she is a sought-after speaker on topics of entrepreneurship, health, and well-being; and she has lectured at venues that include Harvard and New York University. Tara works with the Alliance for a Healthier Generation, an initiative with the American Heart Association and the Clinton Foundation that combats childhood obesity, in order to bring Strala classes to more than 30,000 schools around the United States. She also supports the BOKS program (Build Our Kids' Success), which delivers Strala classes and well-being resources to educators across North America. She lives in New York with her husband Mike Taylor and their daughter, Daisy.